THE PARENT'S GUIDE TO PEDIATRIC DRUGS

THE PARENT'S GUIDE TO PEDIATRIC DRUGS

Ruth McGillis Bindler, R.N., M.S.

Yvonne Tso, R.Ph., M.S.

Linda Berner Howry, R.N., M.S.

HARPER & ROW, PUBLISHERS, New York

Cambridge, Philadelphia, San Francisco, London

Mexico City, São Paulo, Singapore, Sydney

1817

THE PARENT'S GUIDE TO PEDIATRIC DRUGS. Copyright © 1986 by Ruth McGillis Bindler, Yvonne Tso, and Linda Berner Howry. All rights reserved. Printed in the United States of America. No part of this book may be used or reproduced in any manner whatsoever without written permission except in the case of brief quotations embodied in critical articles and reviews. For information address Harper & Row, Publishers, Inc., 10 East 53rd Street, New York, N.Y. 10022. Published simultaneously in Canada by Fitzhenry & Whiteside Limited, Toronto.

FIRST EDITION

Designer: Sidney Feinberg

Library of Congress Cataloging-in-Publication Data

Bindler, Ruth McGillis.
    The parent's guide to pediatric drugs.

    Bibliography; p.
    Includes index.
    1. Pediatric pharmacology—Popular works.   I. Tso,
Yvonne.   II. Howry, Linda Berner.   III. Title.
[DNLM: 1. Drug Therapy—in adolescence—handbooks.
2. Drug Therapy—in infancy & childhood—handbooks.
WS 39 B612p]
RJ560.B56 1986   615.5'8'088054   85-45204
ISBN 0-06-181097-5   86 87 88 89 90 RRD 10 9 8 7 6 5 4 3 2 1
ISBN 0-06-096073·6 (pbk.)   86 87 88 89 90 RRD 10 9 8 7 6 5 4 3 2 1

This book is dedicated to
the parents and children
with whom we have worked.

Contents

Preface   *xi*

PART ONE
SAFEGUARDS FOR GIVING MEDICINES TO YOUR CHILD

1. How Medicines Act in the Child   3

   Absorption   *3*
   Therapeutic Level   *5*
   Metabolism and Excretion   *7*
   Unintended Effects   *8*
   Allergy   *9*
   Pregnancy and Childbirth   *10*
   Breast-feeding   *11*

2. Using Medicines Wisely   13

   Reading and Understanding Labels   *13*
   Medicine Common Sense   *17*
   Cost of Medicines   *18*
   What to Know Before Leaving the Pharmacy   *18*
   Storage of Medicines   *18*
   Medicine Records   *20*
   What Others Caring for Your Child Need to Know About Your
      Child's Medicine   *22*
   How to Transport Medicines When You Travel   *23*

3. Planning the Medicine Experience 25

Planning for Medicine Administration 25
General Developmental Considerations 27

4. Giving Medicines to Your Child 31

By Mouth 31
By Rectum 43
To the Eye 48
For the Ear 55
By the Nose 57
For the Skin and Hair 60
Vaginal Medicines 65

PART TWO
IMMUNIZATIONS

5. Immunizations 71

How Immunizations Work 72
Recommended Immunizations 74

PART THREE
NONPRESCRIPTION MEDICINES

6. Medicines for Fever, Pain, and Inflammation 83

Fever 83
Pain 88
Inflammation 89

7. Vitamins and Minerals 94

Vitamins 97
Minerals 106

8. Medicines for Stomach and Intestinal Discomfort 114

Physiology of the Digestive System 114
Disorders of the Stomach and Intestines and Their Remedies 115

9. Medicines for Breathing Difficulties 141

Physiology of Breathing 141
Disorders of the Respiratory Tract 143
Medicines for Breathing Difficulties 150

10. Medicines for the Eye   160

    Anatomy of the Eye   *160*
    Development of the Eye   *163*
    Common Eye Problems   *164*
    Infections of the Eye   *167*
    Contact Lenses   *169*
    Eye Reactions to Makeup   *170*
    Eye Medicines   *170*
    Other Eye Problems   *177*

11. Medicines for the Ear   178

    Anatomy of the Ear   *178*
    Common Problems of the Outer Ear and Earlobe   *181*
    Infections of the Middle Ear   *183*
    Medicines for the Ear   *184*

12. Medicines for Skin Disorders   187

    Common Skin Disorders   *188*
    Acne Medicines   *197*
    Antibiotics   *199*
    Antiseptics   *200*
    Medicines for Itching   *202*
    Medicines for Parasitic Infections   *203*
    Medicines for Fungal Infections   *204*
    Medicines for Inflammation   *206*
    Diaper Rash Products   *207*
    Sunscreens   *210*

13. Medicines for Weight Control   213

    Overweight   *213*
    Underweight   *214*
    Medicines for Weight Control   *215*

14. Medicines for Menstrual Discomfort   219

    Body Changes Associated with Puberty   *219*
    The Menarche   *220*
    Menstrual Problems   *224*
    Vaginal Products   *227*
    Medications for Menstrual Discomfort   *229*

PART FOUR
COMMON PRESCRIPTION MEDICINES

15. Medicines for Infections   239
    Commonly Prescribed Antibiotics   *240*

16. Medicines for Seizure and Behavioral Control   258
    Commonly Prescribed Medicines   *258*

17. Medicines for the Heart and Lungs   273
    Commonly Prescribed Cardiac and Respiratory Medicines *273*

APPENDIX

1. Table of Common Equivalents and Table of Metric
   Equivalents   286
2. Conversion of Human Temperatures from Fahrenheit to
   Centigrade   287
3. How to Use a Bulb Syringe to Suction an Infant's Nose 288
4. Home First-Aid Supplies   290

Glossary   291
Selected Readings   294
Index   299

Preface

Parents and health care providers have a common aim—caring for children to promote their health and comfort. Medicine plays an integral part in that process, and you as a parent have the right to understand the prescription and nonprescription medicines your child receives— their purpose, how to give them, and possible unintended effects. While there are a number of drug reference books available to you, few specifically address medicines for children. This book answers questions about the pharmacological, physiological, and psychosocial needs of the child.

A child's body often handles medicines differently than an adult's does. Some medicines are used primarily in childhood, while others are not safe for children. Some of the common illnesses necessitate frequent use of certain medicines. A young child may not understand why medicines are given, requiring novel approaches by the parent to obtain cooperation and safely administer medicines. Other developmental needs, both physical and psychosocial, should be considered at various ages.

Medicines are often prescribed by a health care provider. In busy medical offices, hospitals, or pharmacies, you may not receive or fully understand important information about the medicines being given to your child. In addition, you, as a consumer, are frequently exposed to conflicting advice when selecting from the wide variety of nonprescription medicines available for children.

As parents and health care professionals, we understand the difficulty of your task and the confusion you often feel. For this reason we (two nurses and a clinical pharmacist) have written this book.

Part One deals with how your child is different from you and how medicines act in the child's body. There are descriptions of how to approach your child and gain the child's cooperation as well as how to give various types of medications.

Part Two deals with immunizations and why they are important for your child. It includes a schedule of when each immunization should be given. In Part Three the various body systems, which may need nonprescription medicines for the relief of discomfort, are discussed. The anatomy and physiology of the organs and their common ailments are presented, followed by some of the medicines that can be used to treat each body area.

Part Four discusses the common prescription medicines. It helps you understand why the drug is used, how it is given, how it may affect your child, and some of the more common unintended side effects that may occur.

The Bibliography contains information on child care books, and the Glossary offers an explanation of medical terms.

Several terms are used throughout the text to make ideas clearer and to assist in readability. We use the term *health care provider* to refer to the physician, physician's assistant, nurse, nurse practitioner, and pharmacist, since all these individuals provide health care to the child. The term *prescriber* refers to those who we traditionally think of as prescribing, such as doctors, as well as those who have prescriptive authorities under special provisions of the law, such as some nurse practitioners and physicians' assistants.

The terms *medicine, medication,* and *drug* are used throughout this book. They are all synonymous. *Nonprescription* and *over-the-counter* refer to medicines that can be purchased without a prescription in a pharmacy or drugstore.

This book can be of great assistance to parents, but it is not a substitute for the advisory role of the health care provider. If your child is ill and not responding to home care, or if you are uncertain about the cause of an illness, consult a health care provider at once. When you select a nonprescription medicine, consult your pharmacist to gain necessary information about the medicine.

We would like to thank many individuals, particularly those listed here, who have assisted in numerous ways with the writing of this book. Our gratitude goes to the many parents and children who allowed us to photograph them; to our photographers Sidney Cooper, Bil Paul, and

Roy Ramsey for their professional help and suggestions; to Renee LeDoux for her illustrations; to the professionals and parents who carefully read our chapters and gave us valuable insights and suggestions: Major Joyce Shank R.N., U.S. Army; Stan Robinson, M.D.; Kathy Springer, R.N.; Victor Lee, Pharm.D.; Susan and Leonard Griesz; Linda Pregent; Dora McClelland; and Roberta Artzer. We also wish to thank our editors at Harper & Row: Carol Cohen and, especially, Helen Moore for her support and ever-ready assistance. Last but not least, we thank our families, who gave us much support and encouragement in this endeavor.

The information provided in this book about medicines is intended as a general guide for parents and does not constitute all of the information that is available. After careful perusal of the related literature, the authors have used their personal experience and knowledge to select the information of greatest overall importance. This book, then, is meant to be a source of general information that aids parents when choosing nonprescription medicines and when administering medicine to children. It should *not* be used as the only source of medical care or advice but as a supplement to regular contact with a health care provider.

The brand names listed for various medicines serve only as illustrations of common preparations; they are not intended to be complete lists of all available brands, nor do the presence and order of brand names indicate the authors' preferences or recommendations. Every nonprescription and prescription medicine could not be described, so only the more common ones are included.

Carefully consider your child's medical history when administering any medicine. If your child has a chronic condition or receives medicine regularly, seek the direction of your health care provider before changing medicines or adding nonprescription medicine treatment. A child can display individual characteristics in response to medicines. Therefore, you should carefully monitor the treatment of your child. If your child's condition persists, worsens, or changes, seek your health care provider's guidance promptly.

Once again, we emphasize that our aim is not to replace contact with health care providers; we urge you to see them regularly. We wish instead to provide information that can make medicine administration a safer, more knowledgeable, and rewarding experience for you and your child.

PART ONE

*Safeguards
for Giving Medicines
to Your Child*

CHAPTER 1

How Medicines Act in the Child

The child is not simply a small adult with a body that functions like an adult's. While some organs in the young child's body are nearly adultlike in the way they function, others are quite immature until adolescence. Since medicines affect and are affected by many body organs, the maturity of these organs can influence how quickly the medicine gets broken down, eliminated from the body, or achieves its effect. After reading this chapter you will understand some of the ways medicines achieve their effects and realize the importance of checking for specific child-size doses before giving any medicine to your child.

Absorption

In order to achieve the desired effect, a medicine must get into the blood so it can get carried to the part of the body where its effect is needed. Medicines taken by mouth cross into the blood vessels surrounding the stomach and intestines. For the first few months of a child's life, the amounts of acid in the stomach vary and the levels of many digestive substances are low. The different environment in the infant's digestive system can slow, retard, or enhance absorption of medicines. Thus watching for desired and unintended effects is important, especially in the infant. In the child and adolescent, absorption from the stomach and intestines is more predictable.

In general, it is best if oral medicines (those taken by mouth) are given on an empty stomach; this helps absorption. So try to give most medicines thirty minutes before or two hours after feedings. While this is not too difficult with preschoolers or older children, it can be very difficult with infants who are eating frequently. Perhaps you can administer the medicine when your baby awakes and delay the feeding until after diapering, bathing, or playing. See how you manage and check with your health care provider for more guidance. The absorption of a few medicines is not impaired when they are given with food. It may even be helpful to administer those that tend to cause stomach discomfort with a meal, since this may decrease the discomfort. Check with the pharmacist and the descriptions in this book for recommendations about specific medicines. Most medicines need to dissolve in water before they can enter the bloodstream. Giving pills to your child with a generous amount of water or other fluid helps this process, thus facilitating absorption.

When a fast effect is needed or when a medicine is destroyed by stomach fluids, as insulin is, it is given by injection. If it is injected into the fat (subcutaneous) layer by hypodermic injection or the muscle layer by intramuscular injection, the medicine then crosses over into the blood vessels in that area.

The blood flow in infants is less predictable than that of older children, especially during illness. The length of time an injected medicine takes to get absorbed into the circulating blood and achieve its effect is also long and somewhat unpredictable. This is why the baby who is ill and needs treatment quickly is usually hospitalized so that necessary medicines can be administered directly into the bloodstream by intravenous infusion, thus bypassing the need for absorption.

Intravenous infusions, which are placed in veins, can be difficult to administer to young children. The infant has poor circulation on the exterior part of the body, so veins for placement of a needle can be hard to find. You can imagine how small the veins of an infant are, creating difficulty in placing a needle. Although suitable veins are sometimes found in the arms or legs, the veins of the scalp are often best for intravenous infusion in infants. Many parents are frightened when they see an infusion into their baby's head; knowing that this is a normal place for intravenous infusion can allay fear. The small amount of hair shaved to make the vein visible for puncture gradually grows back when the infusion is discontinued.

A few medicines are administered by ways other than oral or injection. Some are inhaled and cross into the blood vessels in the lungs; some melt under the tongue or inside the cheeks and pass into the blood vessels in the mouth; some are applied directly to the skin; and some are placed in the rectum, where they pass into the blood vessels in the lower intestines.

Occasionally a medicine does not even need to get absorbed into the blood to be effective. When you put an antiseptic on your child's cut finger, it prevents infection in the cut by its presence there. Although a little of the antiseptic may be absorbed into the bloodstream, it achieves its effect not by the small amount circulating through the blood but rather by the larger amount present at the cut.

The skin of babies is thin and permeable, allowing substances to pass readily through it and into the body. It is also sensitive and may react with a rash to medicines and other substances. While the skin of preschoolers and school-age children is thicker, truly adult skin is not in place until oil and sweat glands become fully active in adolescence. Avoid skin medicines unless there is a specific indication, and use only preparations intended for skin application on your child's skin; the tendency for substances to be absorbed through the skin puts the child at risk if potentially harmful substances are applied and absorbed into the body.

In general, the least predictability in absorption rate of medicines exists in the infant and very young child. If a medicine, either prescription or nonprescription, does not appear to be achieving the desired effect or is causing unintended effects in your child, contact your health care provider for advice.

When medicine is manufactured into tablets, liquids, or other forms, it is mixed with other substances, and these can slow down or speed up absorption. The same medicine, manufactured by different drug companies, may be mixed with different substances. Sometimes this is the difference between the usually more expensive name-brand medicine and the usually less expensive generic medicine. Ask your pharmacist which is better. You can often save money by using a generic medicine, but you need to know that it gets absorbed with enough strength and speed to be effective.

Therapeutic Level

The therapeutic level is the amount or dose of a drug adequate to cause the desired effects but low enough to avoid unintended or side effects. Doses to achieve the therapeutic level are recommended based on your child's age, weight, or body surface area. Body surface area measurement is obtained when your health care provider calculates the ratio of your child's height to weight. This measurement of body surface area is important because it gives a clue about how the inside of the body is functioning—how much blood and other fluids the child has, how effectively the kidneys get rid of waste products, and how metabolism is functioning. Since all these functions are critical in how the body handles medicines, health care providers often use body surface area to calculate how much medicine to prescribe, finding it a more accurate method than looking at height or weight alone. A three-year-old who is 35 inches tall and weighs 25 pounds may handle a certain medicine differently from another three-year-old who is 40 inches tall and weighs 40 pounds. Nonprescription medicines are usually labeled with a recommended dose for children of various ages. This dose is based on the average child of that age. If your child is substantially larger or smaller than the average child of the same age, contact the pharmacist to be certain the dose on the label is correct for your child.

In addition to height, weight, and age, other factors influence the amount of medicine your child needs to achieve the therapeutic level. Some medicines are stored in body fat, so that the infant or preschooler who has a small amount of body fat requires a smaller dose. The medicines that are not stored in body fat are dissolved and carried in the liquid or water part of the body. While less of the infant's body weight is comprised of fat, more is comprised of water than in the adult. Sixty percent of the adult body weight is water, while 80 to 85 percent of the infant's body weight is water. You've probably already deduced that the young child needs a larger per-weight dose of water-soluble medicine to be effective than does the adult. Several antibiotics are examples of water-soluble medicines. You should be able to see that you cannot use prescription medicines prescribed for you or another child, adjust the dosage, and give them to your infant for a similar illness. Even if it is the correct medicine, you will not know if half the adult dose is too large to be safe or too small to be effective for the child.

For many medicines, it is important to maintain the therapeutic level for a certain period of time. For example, if the level of an antibiotic falls below the therapeutic level, the bacteria will begin to multiply again, and if the level of phenobarbital falls in the epileptic, a seizure may occur. Medicines such as these must be taken on the prescribed schedule. Other medicines, such as vitamins, may be taken whenever it is convenient during the day, even at a different time each day; they will still be effective.

Some medicines are taken only while symptoms of illness are present. Aspirin, for example, is taken to treat a fever only while the child has a fever. But other medicines are taken regularly to prevent illness—aspirin to treat arthritis, phenobarbital for the epileptic, and insulin for the diabetic, to name a few. Still others are given for a definite period of time: for example, antibiotics for treatment of an infection are commonly given for ten days. In this case it is important to give the antibiotic for the total time prescribed. Even if the child appears better in a day or two, continue to give the antibiotic so that the small numbers of bacteria still in the body cannot grow again and cause future infections or other illness, such as rheumatic fever.

Metabolism and Excretion

The chemical changes occurring in the body are known collectively as metabolism. When most medicines enter the body, they are perceived as foreign substances and are broken down, usually by enzymes produced in the liver. This breakdown process is necessary to transform medicines into their chemical components the body can deal with. While part of the medicine circulates to achieve its desired effect, some of it is being changed in form so it can be eliminated. This breakdown process is faster for some medicines than others. When it occurs quickly and a steady therapeutic level in the blood is needed to treat a problem, as is the case with most antibiotics, several doses of the drug must be taken regularly throughout the day. On the other hand, a medicine that is metabolized slowly can be taken less often, such as phenobarbital, which is taken once or twice daily, since the therapeutic level remains steady for long periods.

The infant does not produce large amounts of liver enzymes, so excretion of medicines can be slowed. Organ immaturity in premature and young infants makes them less able to break down and eliminate medicine, and so they are at greater risk of developing toxic effects. For this reason, if you see a change in behavior in your baby who is taking medicine, report this to your health care provider. Make sure your health care provider knows all the medicines your child is taking. It may be that liver enzymes are being used to break down one medicine, and adding another one to the body can overtax the breakdown ability.

Once a medicine is broken down by liver enzymes, it can be eliminated from the body. Most medicines are excreted in the urine, so kidney function is important. The infant under one year has immature kidneys, so medicines are not eliminated as quickly as in the older child. If the medicine continues to be given regularly, it may build up in the body, causing unintended effects, unless the dose is altered. Babies receiving more than one medicine have an even harder time eliminating these medicines and their waste products and are even more at risk for experiencing unintended effects. So once again, caution is urged with any infant receiving medicines, especially for a prolonged period of time. Remember to tell your health care provider *all* medicines the baby has taken recently when being examined or treated.

The kidneys mature rapidly, so that babies age one to two years are able to eliminate most medicines readily. Infants should urinate six to eight times daily, with this number decreasing somewhat in the toddler and preschooler. If your child begins to urinate very frequently, decreases the number of urinations, or stops urinating totally, see your health care provider promptly. The buildup of medicine waste products in the child who is taking medicine and not urinating regularly can be dangerous. Drinking extra water or other fluids helps ensure that broken-down medicines get eliminated more easily.

Unintended Effects

As you can imagine, while a medicine is traveling through the blood, it has access to a number of body parts in addition to the area where it achieves its desired effect. It may act on some of these areas and create unintended or side effects. Sometimes an antibiotic causes nausea or changes the normal bacteria in the intestines and causes diarrhea. Some medicines cause dizziness. The aim is to reach the therapeutic level: a high enough dose to be effective but low enough to minimize unintended effects. With some medicines this is easy to manage, while with others it is very difficult. At any rate, when you administer any medicine to your child, be alert for unintended effects. Sometimes common ones are listed on the container, but not always. If you have questions consult your health care provider. If the unintended effects are making your child uncomfortable, report them to your health care provider, who may be able to recommend a different medicine with fewer unintended effects. And whenever you are given a prescription for your child, ask if there are common unintended effects for which you can be alert.

Allergy

An allergy or a hypersensitivity to a medicine or other substance can be a serious matter. The body perceives the substance as foreign and sets up a strong reaction, such as swelling of various body parts, profuse itching, hives (skin welts), skin rash, or wheezing (noisy breaths). Rapid, severe allergy is called anaphylaxis and can even lead to death. If a child has had an allergic reaction to a medicine, that medicine should not be taken again, for it may lead to a more severe reaction the second time. If your child is allergic to a medicine, carefully record its name, the dosage received, date, and effects, and relay these to any health care provider. Some medicines are chemically similar to others, so that if a child is allergic to one, the related medicines should also be avoided. For example, children allergic to one sulfa-containing medicine should not receive other medicines with this ingredient, and those with penicillin allergy may be allergic to related medicines, such as ampicillin. In addition, it is possible to be allergic to one of the substances used in the preparation of a medicine and not the medicine itself. For example, some children are allergic to a red dye that is used in the coating on some tablets. In such cases, a different preparation of the same medicine may be substituted. These allergic responses also need to be recorded and reported to any health care provider. We cannot predict who will have allergic reactions, but it seems that if other family members have allergies to certain medicines or other substances, the child is more likely to manifest allergy, even though it may be to a different substance.

Many people confuse allergies with unintended effects. Remember that an unintended effect occurs as a medicine acts on a part of the body other than where it achieves its desired effect. Examples include diarrhea in response to an antibiotic or hard stools with iron ingestion. These are not allergic reactions and should not be called that. If unintended effects are experienced and a health care provider is told it was an allergy, your child could be deprived of that medicine in the future when it is the best treatment for a serious illness. For this reason, when you state that your child has an allergy to a medicine, a health care provider may ask you what happened when it was administered. If your child experiences uncomfortable side effects, perhaps a different form, brand, or dosage of the medicine will work better.

Rashes in response to medicines may or may not indicate an allergic reaction. A rash may be indicative of an allergy to a medicine, but sometimes medicines produce a rash as an unintended effect. Ask the health care provider whether your child's rash indicates allergy or a side effect and whether it is safe for the child to take the medicine in the future.

Pregnancy and Childbirth

The effect of medicines on your child can start even before birth. Nearly everyone is aware of the tragedy that occurred in the 1960s when many women who were treated with the tranquilizer thalidomide during pregnancy gave birth to infants with deformed arms and legs. More recently, some adolescent girls whose mothers were treated with diethylstilbestrol (DES) during pregnancy have developed vaginal adenocarcinoma, a cancer. The list of drugs known to affect the fetus is quite long now, including, among others, tetracycline, which inhibits bone growth and damages tooth enamel; aspirin, which causes bleeding; and tobacco smoke, which causes low-birth-weight babies. Recently the effects of alcohol on the fetus have been well documented, including facial abnormalities and mental retardation. The drug Bendectin, commonly administered to decrease nausea and vomiting in early pregnancy, has been withdrawn from the market after its use was connected with an increase in pyloric stenosis, a stomach abnormality in newborns. In short, one wonders if any medicine is safe to take in pregnancy. Obviously it is better to err on the side of caution, so the use of medicines during pregnancy should be kept to a minimum.

You cannot assume that nonprescription medicines are less powerful and therefore safe; keep in mind that even aspirin affects the fetus. The best policy is to stop the use of all medicines about three months before attempting pregnancy. If you are on a medicine that must be taken, such as insulin or an antiseizure drug, continue taking it but inform your physician of your desire to become pregnant so that any necessary regulation can occur.

Many substances not packaged as pills act as medicines in the body. Tobacco smoke, alcohol, and many illegal street drugs have known effects on the fetus; caffeine and artificial sweeteners have possible but not proved effects. Abstinence from these substances is best; if this is not possible, decrease your intake to the smallest amount possible.

What happens if you really need a medicine during pregnancy? Talk to your health care provider, since there is usually something that can be used to treat an illness that is believed to be relatively safe. Since aspirin is to be avoided, acetaminophen for an occasional ache can usually be used. Check with your health care provider before taking other medicines, even nonprescription products.

Medicines used during childbirth can also affect the newborn. Parents have become more knowledgeable about the process of labor and delivery in recent years and often make informed choices about medication use for childbirth. Methods of pain control such as relaxation and breathing techniques have decreased the need for medicine. Smaller doses and different administration techniques are used when medication is necessary, to minimize the effects on the alertness of the newborn.

Breast-feeding

Just as the fetus is exposed to medicines taken by the pregnant woman, so is the infant exposed to medicines taken by the nursing mother. One medicine may be present in minimal amounts in breast milk, while another may appear in a higher concentration in the milk than in the mother's blood. The amount of medicine excreted in breast milk depends on a number of factors, such as the dosage taken by the mother, the time it is taken, and the properties of the medicine, including how quickly it is broken down and excreted, its degree of solubility, its pH, and how much it attaches itself to body proteins.

In addition, an infant can safely be exposed to some medicines, while others may be harmful. One is quickly metabolized and excreted, while another is more slowly broken down. Slow metabolism of a drug poses a greater threat when the nursing mother takes a medicine over a period of time, since it can accumulate in the infant and possibly cause toxic effects.

It is best for the mother to minimize her medication intake while she is breast-feeding. An occasional analgesic dose of acetaminophen probably has minimal effect on the infant. But medicines used to dry secretions during a cold may decrease the milk supply as well. Other substances have the potential to be excreted in breast milk. For example, alcohol and caffeine act as drugs; moderation in intake is recommended.

Before taking either prescription or nonprescription medicines, tell your health care provider that you are breast-feeding and then watch your infant carefully to see if there are any changes in behavior due to medicine effects. Many Poison Control Centers provide information on medicine effects on the breast-fed baby. If you can, take doses of medicine just after breast-feeding. This will lead to the lowest possible dose in breast milk. Avoid use of long-acting or sustained-release products, since their levels are higher in breast milk.

CHAPTER 2

Using Medicines Wisely

It is important to understand the purpose and methods of administration of all medicines that are prescribed for your child. The physician, nurse, and pharmacist can provide you with information about your child's medicine. Make sure you know what the medicine is for and how it works to relieve your child's symptoms. You should know how to schedule the times the medicine is to be given, how to prepare and measure the medicine, how to give the medicine, how to tell if the medicine is working, and how to watch for any unintended effects. Unintended or side effects can be nausea, diarrhea, vomiting, drowsiness, skin rash, hives, or any other unpleasant symptoms. When you do not fully understand the medicine, contact your doctor, nurse, or pharmacist.

Parents usually select physicians carefully but give less consideration to their pharmacist. Look for a pharmacist who provides you with adequate and understandable information about your prescriptions. When you are selecting a nonprescription medicine, you may need even more assistance, so a knowledgeable pharmacist can direct you to the right medicine and help you save money.

Reading and Understanding Labels

Nonprescription Medicine Labels

In the case of a mild childhood illness for which you do not seek a health care provider's care, you may decide to give your child a nonprescription medicine to increase comfort. Medicines are chemicals and therefore are not harmless. Take great care in choosing any drug. Read labels carefully. Select only medicines recommended by the manufacturer for use by a child. Your pharmacist can provide valuable information concerning nonprescription (over-the-counter) drugs and can answer any questions you may have about them.

Nonprescription medicines are packaged so that you can tell if the drug container has been previously opened.· Medicines may come in double containers, such as a bottle sealed inside a box or canister, tablets inside individual foil containers so you just push the tablets out as you use them, or bottles with a plastic or metal ring around the cap that must be broken when the bottle is first opened. Check all medicines you purchase to make sure these various seals are intact, and do not purchase or use the medicine when you are uncertain about the security of the seal. If the item is packaged in a double container, be sure to read all labels on the outer container before discarding it.

Specific information about a medicine can be obtained from its label. This enables you to understand the contents of the medicine and how to use the drug. The front label usually lists the medicine's name, both generic and trade; the drug's classification (what it does for an illness); the ingredients in milligrams per dosage; and the manufacturer's name.

A generic name is the pharmacological name used for a chemical of a particular structure. This name is decided upon by appointed drug experts and sanctioned by governmental agencies. The trade or brand name is given by the drug company to its particular brand of medicine. It is registered to distinguish it from any other drug company's form of the medicine. On a medicine label, the trade name generally appears first and the generic name follows in smaller print. For example, the trade name Tylenol is listed in large print on the label and the generic name, acetaminophen, is listed in smaller print. By carefully reading these names, you may find that you are buying the same generic drug under several different trade names and at various prices.

The drug's classification tells you what it does. For instance, an antibacterial such as Bacitracin fights germs or bacteria, whereas an antacid such as Mylanta neutralizes stomach acid. The ingredients are listed by the number of milligrams per dose and are usually in order of the highest dose of the active ingredient down to the lowest. Also listed is the total quantity of medicine in the container.

The back or side label tells how much medicine is to be administered for each age or weight group and how often it can be given safely.

Follow these instructions closely to avoid giving your child an overdose of medicine either by giving too large a dose or by giving it too frequently. Warnings such as "harmful if taken internally," "do not use this drug if you have kidney disease," and "keep out of reach of children" are also listed. Some may list drug interaction precautions, for instance, "do not take this product with an antibiotic containing tetracycline." Information on proper storage of the medicine is also found on the label.

Expiration date of the medicine, on the other hand, may appear on the label, at the end of the tube (called the crimp), or on the bottom of the bottle. After this date the medicine's chemical content may be altered by its age. It may not contain the correct potency or it may fail to produce the desired effects. Check the expiration date with each use. Do not use any outdated medicine.

Next to the expiration date appears a series of numbers. This is the manufacturer's lot number. This number identifies when and where a specific batch of medicine was produced. This information becomes important if for some reason there was an error or if it was found that a batch somehow was contaminated and is not safe for use.

Prescription Medicine Labels

A prescription drug label differs from a nonprescription label in a number of ways. Most of the information is typed by your pharmacist, as every prescription is different. Besides the name, address, and telephone number of the pharmacy filling the prescription, a prescription medicine label contains the following information:

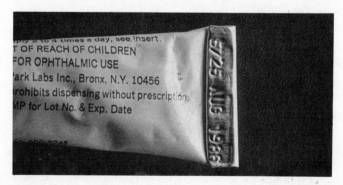

The expiration date of medicine sold in a tube is found at the bottom edge, called the crimp. *(Bil Paul)*

- The date the medicine is issued to you.
- A prescription number that identifies this prescription to the pharmacy; this number helps the pharmacy locate the original prescription if there are any questions regarding the medicine.
- Your child's name and the dosage to be taken, usually listed in household measurements such as teaspoons, or in cubic centimeters if it is a liquid preparation.
- Instructions for how often and how long the medicine is to be taken: "take one teaspoon three times a day for 10 days," for instance.
- The medicine name and the health care provider who prescribed it. The way the medicine name appears on the prescription varies from state to state. Some states require that both the generic and trade names of the

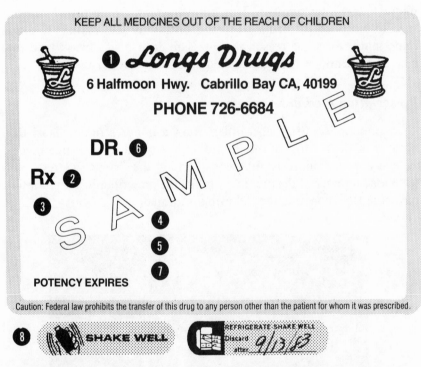

A prescription drug label gives the following information: (1) the name, address, and phone number of the pharmacy dispensing the drug; (2) the prescription number; (3) the name of the person for whom the drug has been prescribed; (4) the name of the medicine; (5) dosage and administration instructions; (6) the name of the doctor who wrote the prescription; (7) special preparation information; (8) applicable warning labels.

medicine be listed. In other states the pharmacy lists the medicine as your doctor prescribed it, so if a trade name was used, that will be listed. If, however, you request the generic form of the drug, both the generic and trade name ordered should appear on the label.

- Preparation, storage, and warning information, such as "shake well before using," "keep refrigerated," "do not operate heavy machinery while taking this medication," or "keep out of direct sunlight" may appear on the label or on colored stickers on the container.
- Certain medicines are categorized by federal law as controlled substances. These medicines are not to be used or transferred to any other persons. A warning label usually appears on the bottle that reads, "Federal law prohibits transfer of this medication to other persons."

Medicine Common Sense

As stated previously, you need to understand how medicine works in your child's body before you administer it. This is especially significant for nonprescription drugs, since with them you are making the decision about what to administer. Some television commercials and magazine and newspaper advertisements about nonprescription drugs may confuse the consumer about the medicine. For example, you see a new product advertised as a revolutionary painkiller, but when you read the label, you discover it is a common pain relief agent, packaged under a different company's new trade name. This is not misrepresentation, because this manufacturer may not have produced this generic drug before or the proportion of ingredients in the product may indeed be different from that in other existing brands. It is misleading, because the medicine is not a new discovery but one produced by other pharmaceutical companies. So always read the package label before selecting the product you wish to purchase. Be sure to check the generic name of the medicine and not just the trade name. If you have any questions or doubts, ask your pharmacist.

Nonprescription medicines come in various strengths and sizes. Do not be confused by equivalent measures in various products. One may be advertised as having a full gram of strength and another as having 1000 milligrams. These measures are the same. Refer to Appendix 1 for a table of equivalents to assist you.

Read the label of nonprescription medicines to discover if they contain any substance to which your child may be allergic. Check the quantity of each ingredient. Several products may be designed to do the same thing. However, one may be more effective than others for your child for a particular illness due to the different proportions of various ingredients. The pharmacist can assist you in making these decisions.

Cost of Medicines

Since the cost of medical care and medicines is continually rising, it pays to be an informed consumer. In most states you can call any pharmacy and compare the price of a prescription or a nonprescription medicine prior to purchase. Costs do vary among pharmacies. In some states you can request the generic form of a prescription drug, which is usually cheaper and in most cases is equally effective. Your pharmacist can inform you about the action of the generic drug in comparison with the prescribed brand of medicine. Some states require that the physician decide if a generic medicine can be substituted for the one prescribed. If this is your state's law, discuss with the prescriber if a generic form of the medicine can be used.

What to Know Before Leaving the Pharmacy

When you leave your pharmacy, you should feel confident that the medicine you purchased, be it prescription or nonprescription, is what you need for your child's illness. This means understanding the drug's desired action, how much to give, and how often each dose is to be given. Do you know how to administer and store the medicine? Do you have an accurate measuring device if the medicine is a liquid? More detailed information about what you should know before giving medicine is found in Chapter 3, under Planning for Medicine Administration.

Storage of Medicines

Ask your health care provider or read the label of a drug to learn of any special storage instructions for the medicine you buy. There are some general principles you should know. Any medicine you bring into your household should have child-resistant caps if your children are of preschool age or younger. Accidental ingestion of drugs by children is not uncommon. When closing bottles with child-resistant caps, make sure the locking mechanism has engaged. If the mechanism has not locked the bottle, it will open like a screw-type top. Keeping the tops of liquid medicines clean helps the locking mechanism engage properly and prevents the growth of germs on the neck of the bottle and cap.

Keep all medicines in locked cabinets, boxes, or other locked storage devices. Bathroom medicine cabinets or any other cabinets are not satisfactory for storing medicines unless they are securely locked. Any type of box, such as a fishing tackle box, with a padlock or other type of child-proof lock attached, can serve as a safe medicine cabinet.

Your storage box or area should be dry, since moisture can alter the chemical composition of a drug. Extreme temperatures, either freezing cold or high heat, can also alter the chemical nature of liquid, tablet, or capsule forms of medicines, so your locked box or area should be maintained at a temperature of 55°F to 75°F. Avoid keeping your medicines in direct sunlight, such as on a windowsill. Amber-colored bottles provide adequate protection against sunlight, so medicines sensitive to light usually come in these containers.

Keep all liquid medicines in their original bottles. Certain liquid medicines, such as antibiotics, and some rectal medicines may require refrigeration. When you have a liquid medicine that requires refrigeration, put the bottle in the very back of the top shelf of the refrigerator and keep all other liquids in your locked area. Placing the refrigerated medicine in the back on a high shelf serves two purposes. First, the temperature variations are less than on the shelves of the door, and second, a child is less likely to be tempted to take the medicine bottle if it is less visible.

Since rectal suppositories are not usually sold in child-resistant jars or boxes, be extra careful about keeping them where your child is unable to gain access to them. Some parents have found that if medicines like suppositories are placed in a labeled, opaque, plastic, resealable container, they are less visible to the small child and thereby less tempting.

Always store tablets and capsules in their original containers; when removed, their names and dosages are easily forgotten. If you place several different kinds of pills in a single container, it is easy to confuse them, especially if they are similar in appearance. Never give your child a medicine that you cannot positively identify. Fatal mistakes can be and have been made.

Most eye, ear, nose, and skin preparations come in containers that are not child-resistant, so you must take special care to lock them up. Even antiseptic skin cleansing products must be locked away. Read the label or package insert to see if they are harmful if taken internally (eaten). Remember that most of these products can be harmful if they come in contact with the eyes or mucous membranes of the mouth, nose, or genital region.

It is a good idea to go through your locked medicine area periodically and discard outdated medicines. The contents should be removed from the bottles and not just thrown into the wastebasket, where the child can find them. Pour liquids down the drain and flush tablets and capsules down the toilet.

Your home may be safe for children, but what about those of your neighbors, grandparents, and friends? Small children have opportunities to explore other households and can get into medicines there as easily as in their own homes. Take the case of the four- and two-year-old who were visiting their grandmother. She had a large chewable chocolate-flavored laxative bar in the drawer of the bathroom sink vanity. The children found the laxative and ate the entire bar without telling anyone. The two-year-old almost died from the resulting severe diarrhea and dehydration. Don't let this happen to your child.

When you have guests visiting or spending the night, make sure your child does not have access to purses or suitcases that may contain medicines. Often times the elderly have medicines stored in containers without child-resistant caps because they are unable to get them open due to weakness or disease conditions such as arthritis. Remind your guests to lock all suitcases with medication in them.

Medicine Records

Your health care provider keeps a record of all your visits. Included in this record is an account of all medicines prescribed for your child. Most parents do not have access to these records. In a mobile society it is not uncommon to utilize several health facilities while a child is growing up. Thus there may not be one single record with the child's complete medical history. Occasionally it may be necessary when your child becomes an adult to find out if a certain medicine was taken in childhood. If your health care provider has already retired from practice, it may be difficult to find this information. Several years from now you will not remember the names and dates of the medicines your child has received. Thus you can see the value of keeping your own medical records. It is very simple to do and may be an invaluable source of information for your child in the future.

Keep your child's immunization records up to date, because they are required by most nurseries, day-care centers, preschools, and elementary schools prior to your child's admission. This is done to control communicable diseases. The immunization record is required for international travel to most foreign countries. These records are given to you by the health care provider when your child is first immunized. Do not lose these cards or papers. Take them with you every time your child receives an immunization, so the record can be updated. It is also helpful to keep a duplicate record in case you lose the original. Just copy the date, type of immunization, amount of medicine given, and name of the physician or clinic where the immunization was given. You should also record any reaction your child experienced to the immunizations. If you make a duplicate and ever lose the original, you will know where and when the child was immunized. Your clinic or health care provider's office should also have a copy of the immunization history for your child.

An effective method of keeping a record of your child's other medicines is to use a separate notebook for each child. It is also helpful

Aaron's Record

DATE	ILLNESS	MEDICINE	DOSAGE	RESULTS
Sept 18, 1985	Awoke complaining of R+ear pain (right ear infection)	Amoxicillin	250 mg (1tsp.) 3 times / day	no problems
Sept 25, 1985	Awoke crying. both ears hurting (infection in both ears)	changed SEPTRA	Two tsp. 2 times / day	28th Sept. Complaining of upset stomach and diarrhea, ears still hurt
Sept 28, 1985	Reaction from large dose Septra NOT AN ALLERGY Ear infection remains	changed CECLOR ®	250 mg (1tsp) 3 times / day	Finished Medication ears are OK

A sample notebook used to keep a child's medicine record.

if the notebook is small enough to fit inside a purse or pocket, and it should be started for each child at birth.

The medicine record can be set up in a variety of ways, but it should contain the following information:

- the date—including the day, month, and year
- the illness—what your child was treated for
- the medicine—what you gave or what was prescribed by the health care provider (the medicine name can be obtained from the prescription or medicine label)
- the dosage—how much you gave and how often the medicine was given; in the case of an antibiotic, note if the full course was completed
- the results—record the child's response to the medicine: did the child get better? Were unintended effects experienced? Was there any allergy to the medicine?

If your child is allergic to a medicine, write its name, the date the allergy was first noted, and how the allergy was manifested on the front inside cover. It is also helpful to write in this book if your child had any childhood illnesses, such as mumps or chickenpox, and when these illnesses occurred. With this information you will never have to rely on memory for this valuable data. It is very difficult to remember what a child had ten to twenty years after the fact, especially if you have more than one child.

What Others Caring for Your Child Need to Know About Your Child's Medicine

You may not always be the one to give medicine to your child. It is necessary for those responsible for him or her to understand how and when to give the medicine. It is best to write down the time, medicine name, and dosage. If it is a liquid medicine, show the caretaker who gives the medicine how to measure it, using the measuring device. Explain how your child takes the medicine and ask the caretaker to write down when the medicine was given. This serves as a reminder to the caretaker and gives you a record of the medicine dosage. If rectal, eye, nasal, or ear medicines are to be given, you need to evaluate whether the caretaker is competent to give the medicine. If your child is cared for away from home and is taking medicine that needs refrigeration, be sure to check on whether the facility has a refrigerator.

If your child is in school, medicine is usually dispensed from the school nurse's office. The teacher may also give the medicine. Be sure to check on medicine policies with the school where your child is enrolled. It is best to know these policies before an illness occurs.

How to Transport Medicines When You Travel

Medicine should be transported in its original container. In some states this is the law. When the directions are on the container, you'll never wonder what the medicine is or how often to give it.

Tablets and capsules can be transported with relative ease. If you have young children, remember to keep the medicine locked up, such as in the carry-on baggage to which you have direct access. Thus the medicine is available when you need it and won't be lost if your luggage is missing, especially if you travel by plane. Your purse is not a safe place, because it cannot be locked and many children love to explore.

Liquid medications present problems when traveling because they often spill or require refrigeration. To see if tablets or capsules can be substituted, when you purchase the medicine inform your pharmacist that you will be traveling. Tablets can be crushed, and the contents of capsules can be mixed with a small amount of food, such as jelly, to disguise the taste. See page 33 for more specific information.

If you must travel with liquid medication, you can prevent spilling by placing a plastic wrap tightly over the top of the bottle before attaching the cap. Another safeguard is to place masking tape around the closed cap.

Liquid antibiotics that require refrigeration can present quite another problem when traveling. You can carry the liquid antibiotic on ice. Place the bottle of medicine inside a resealable plastic container or bag. Make sure this container has no holes. Now place the container that has the medicine bottle in it inside another container and fill it with ice. You will have to check it frequently to replace the ice and dump out the water. Airlines will often place a bottle of medicine in their refrigerator for you or will give you ice while in flight.

For short trips a liquid medicine that requires refrigeration generally can be left unrefrigerated for about one hour. But keep in mind the actual weather conditions. If both the temperature and humidity are high and you are traveling in an unairconditioned vehicle, the medicine's chemical composition may be affected. Placing the bottle in an insulated freezer bag helps maintain a better environment for the liquid medicine. If you are uncertain whether the liquid medicine needs refrigeration or for how long you can keep it out of the refrigerator, consult a pharmacist.

Running Out of Medicine

If you forget to bring your child's medicine when traveling in your own state, especially if the trip is unexpected, go to a pharmacy and explain your predicament. The pharmacist can call your prescriber and try to find a way to accommodate your need. Prescriptions may not be transferrable from state to state, so have this prescription filled in the state where the health care provider practices. Each state governs whether they will accept prescriptions from health care prescribers in other states.

CHAPTER 3

Planning the Medicine Experience

This chapter helps parents become more knowledgeable about preparing medicines for a sick child so they can correctly give medicine while making the experience less traumatic. A positive medicine experience allows the child to cooperate and prevents the feeling that medicine is given as a punishment.

Planning for Medicine Administration

First you must establish the medicine administration schedule. Knowledge of the drug's chemical makeup and its desired action in your child's body allowed your health care provider to set a prescribed schedule. Verify the schedule so you know when to administer the drug. For example, if the medicine is to be taken three time daily, clarify whether this means every eight hours, at mealtimes, or at other intervals throughout the day. Chapter 1 explains that the times of administration can be critical for some medicine to work correctly. Plan the times you give the medicine to facilitate the drug's action and also to fit into your child's daily schedule as well as possible.

Whoever gives the medicine—you, another adult, or your child if old enough—should wash her or his hands prior to medicine preparation. This helps prevent the introduction of germs into the medicine. Assemble any needed equipment, such as the medicine bottle, oral syringe, or cup with your child's favorite fluid. Reread the medicine label to assure yourself that you are giving the right medicine to the right child in the right amount. Prescription bottles often look alike, which contributes to making errors.

Regardless of the child's age or the type of medicine being given, make certain that the child is safe during the administration. This means that the child is positioned on a surface to prevent falls. Infants have fallen from changing tables, out of infant seats, and from beds. Gather all the necessary equipment and medicine and have it within your reach before you begin to give the medicine. Organize everything so you do not have to turn your back on the child. If you must turn around, always have your hand on the child's abdomen so you can feel the child's movement. To prevent injuries if the child resists, enlist the aid of another person or use an appropriate restraining device.

How you react to a situation clues your child to react to the same situation. If you are upset about an experience, your facial expressions and body language relay your feelings, even if you sound reassuring. If you taste a medicine and make a face, you may have difficulty convincing your child that the medicine is palatable. Past experiences with medicine also influence the way the child cooperates with the current medicine regimen. For example, if the last medicine you gave your four-year-old was bad-tasting, it will not be easy to convince the child that this medicine is different, especially if it happens to be the same color.

Take a positive approach. You know the medicine must be taken, but if you ask, "Would you like to take your medicine now?", you are giving the option to choose not to take it. Instead give the child choices that can be made, like which fluid to drink following the medicine.

Do not bribe a child with toys or money to take medicine. You may get the child to take the medicine now, but a reward will be expected in the future. It is better to use fluids to counteract a medicine's bad taste, offer to read a story, or award stars on a chart when the medicine is taken.

Always be honest in your description of procedures or tastes of medicines. Honesty reinforces the child's trust and belief in what you do and say. If the medication tastes bad, you might say, "This does not taste good but the medicine is necessary to make you well. You can have some fruit juice to take the taste away after you have taken all of it." Always stress that medicine is given either to make you well, to prevent you from getting sick, or to prevent symptoms of disease. Children should learn that medicine is given for a specific purpose and should not be taken if it is not necessary.

General Developmental Considerations

The Infant (Birth to One Year)

The period in life from birth to one year of age is one not only of rapid growth but of great intellectual development for the infant. The child is learning to control body movements and gaining trust in the environment.

An infant, obviously does not understand a verbal explanation of a procedure. However, comfort and positive feelings are gained upon hearing the familiar parent's voice. So during any medication experience, talk or sing to your child. This will probably make the experience less frightening. If the child is having something painful done (for example, a nurse or doctor giving an immunization injection), the sound of your voice lets your presence be known.

Following any medicine experience, holding and cuddling the infant promotes feelings of security and love. A pacifier also may quiet and soothe an infant during and following an injection or other painful procedure.

The Toddler (One to Three Years Old)

Since your toddler has now learned the magic word no and uses it in response to every question, it is important to be positive in your approach. Don't give choices. For example, do not ask, "Would you like to take your medicine now?" Instead it is better to say, "Here is your medicine to take now."

Even though this age group now understands basic instructions, their comprehension of events is limited. The toddler is egocentric and only wants to know about what is happening to him or her and not about others. Therefore there is minimal benefit from seeing a brother or sister receiving medicines.

The concept of time is limited, and most toddlers do not understand morning, afternoon, today, or tomorrow. Explaining things too far in advance is frightening to children this age, so it is a better practice to inform a toddler about medicine time immediately before you give it. However, if your child asks about his medicine time, explain time in terms that can be understood. For instance, "After you eat your lunch and have your nap, Mommy will give you your eyedrops."

Toddlers are also unable to understand fully what causes things to happen. For example, if your toddler gets disciplined for running out into the street when you arrive at the health care provider's office or clinic for a measles immunization, the child may think that the injection is also part of the punishment. Emphasize that medicine is not a punishment. Avoid calling a child bad or naughty when she or he is uncooperative about medicine administration. Instead give praise when there is cooperation.

If a medicine experience is stressful, provide a stress-reducing play session. Pounding toys, such as a hammer and peg bench, and balls can assist the toddler in getting over stressful situations. The banging and throwing motions take out aggression and show the child how to handle frustrations in a socially acceptable manner.

Since the toddler has gained control of the body and fine motor movements, and because of a relentless curiosity, accidental poisonings are common. Medicine bottles and tubes hold a special fascination. Toddlers have been known to drink whole bottles of medicine or smear a tube of medication all over themselves. For this reason all medicines should be placed securely out of their reach in locked containers. Teach your child not to eat anything unless an adult is asked first. Teach your toddler that vitamins, iron tablets, and refrigerated medicines can be harmful. Post the Poison Control Center phone number near your phone in case of accidental ingestions. (For information on how to use syrup of ipecac, see p. 139).

The Preschooler (Three to Six Years Old)

Your three- to six-year-old preschooler seems to be overflowing with new language skills. Although many words are spoken, the knowledge of their meaning may still be limited. Thus the preschooler may have difficulty expressing feelings verbally but will do better in imaginative play or with freehand drawings. For example, a five-year-old boy disliked an oral medicine he was receiving while hospitalized. He would take the medicine grudgingly but never told his mother why he was upset. The medicine did not taste bad. In play with miniature hospital equipment, he used the nurse doll and baby doll and spit the medicine in their faces. Other play with dolls demonstrated his anger at a new baby brother who had just been brought home. This play showed the hostility and anger he was unable to express verbally, because two days after the baby came home, this preschooler was hospitalized. He saw the medicine as the reason he had to stay in the hospital and his new baby brother as taking his place at home.

You may also gain insight into your preschooler's feelings by asking the child to draw a picture and then asking for an explanation about what is happening in the picture. The preschool child's understanding of where the body parts are and how they function is vague. Preschoolers may think, for example, that what is inside the body will fall out when the body is cut. This is why a plastic adhesive strip placed over a wound provides consolation; the cut is covered and the body is intact again.

The preschooler fears body intrusion, especially in the genital region. This child is egocentric like the toddler and does not benefit from seeing other children take medicine. He only cares about how it feels to him.

The School-Age Child (Six to Twelve Years Old)

School age is a time of increased understanding. This child understands explanations and has a curiosity about the body and how it functions. Use explanations and drawings to contribute to the understanding of illness and the necessity for medicine.

The peer group has significant influence on thoughts and ideas. Although the family is important, the chief concern is with the peer group's views and acceptance. Anything that the school-ager views as different from the peer group is perceived as threatening to the relationship with the group.

Anxiety and frustrations can be verbalized by children in this age group. However, they do rid themselves of a lot of stress through activities such as running and other outdoor sports. If your child has to stay in bed because of an illness or injury, you may notice increased irritability due to the child's inability to get rid of stress. If the illness will permit, Velcro dart and ball games as well as simply tossing a bean bag or ball into a wastebasket can help get rid of tensions.

The Adolescent (Twelve to Eighteen Years Old)

Somewhere near the end of school age and the beginning of adolescence, your child experiences puberty. Hormonal influences cause changes in physical appearance and also directly affect the emotions causing mood swings. Each child responds to these changes differently. The adolescent's task becomes one of accepting him- or herself and establishing his or her own identity. Sensitivity and understanding by the parent will assist the child through these times.

Most teens have a good understanding of the human body and its functions from school science courses. Most teens can be responsible for their own medicine administration. Information on how the drug is to be taken, why it is needed, and how it works in the body must be given. Adolescents are capable of understanding the complete details of an illness and how the medicine influences the course of the disease. The adolescent needs to know if the medicine produces unintended effects so that he or she does not simply elect not to take the medicine if these occur.

School-age children and adolescents can be exposed to alcohol and illicit drugs. They must be made aware that these substances can interact with prescription and nonprescription medicines, producing undesirable or even fatal effects. If you feel uncomfortable about discussing these issues with your child, or you feel your child does not feel free to discuss this issue with you, contact your health care provider. This individual usually can discuss these issues with your child in a nonthreatening and nonjudgmental manner.

CHAPTER 4

Giving Medicines to Your Child

As a parent, you are the best judge of your child's behavior and mood. From your observations and understanding of your child, you gain her or his trust and cooperation. This chapter offers information and ideas on giving your child medicines that will assist you in making the medicine experience positive.

By Mouth

This is the most common way to give medicine to a child. It is called the oral route by health care providers. Medicines that are taken by mouth are available as liquids, tablets, and capsules.

Liquid Medicine

A child under five usually cannot swallow a pill and may get the tablet caught in the throat, cutting off the air supply to the lungs. For this reason liquid medicines are usually used for young children. Liquid medicine has the active drug dissolved or suspended in a fluid. Flavoring agents are sometimes added to disguise the medicine's taste.

Liquid medicines include elixers, suspensions, and drops. An elixir contains just enough alcohol to dissolve the drug contents so that they can be mixed with water to form a solution. They are clear and usually do not require shaking to mix the drug into solution. Oral suspensions are cloudy in appearance and are shaken prior to administration to ensure that the drug is evenly distributed in the liquid. The ingredients

31

tend to settle to the bottom of the bottle upon standing. If this happens, unless the bottle is shaken, your child does not get a sufficient dosage of the drug in the beginning and gets too much toward the bottom of the bottle.

If your child has allergies or is diabetic, it is important to check the compounds listed on the medication label of any nonprescription drugs you plan to give and to check with your physician or pharmacist about prescription drugs. This prevents the allergic child from inadvertently getting a substance that causes an allergic reaction.

Liquid medicines in a sugar solution contain large amounts of sugar, which may affect a diabetic child's blood sugar control. If a liquid preparation contains sugar, it is helpful if your child rinses the mouth or brushes the teeth after taking the medicine. This achieves two things: first, it cleans the mouth of the sugar that could cause tooth decay, and second, it may help rid the mouth of a medication's bad taste. However, if the medicine has been given to treat the mouth or throat for a local effect, such as with nystatin for thrush, do not rinse the mouth or brush the teeth following the taking of the medicine.

Measuring Liquid Medicines

Medicine should be measured carefully and accurately to ensure that your child receives the correct dosage. Most prescriptions use the household measurement system, which measures volume by the drop, teaspoon, tablespoon, cup, and glass. You may on occasion see the metric system used. The basic units are the liter and milliliter (or cubic centimeter) for measuring a volume of liquid.

In 1903 the American Medical Association stated that one teaspoon was to contain 5 cubic centimeters (cc) or milliliters (ml) to measure liquid medicine. Thus, if your physician prescribes for your child 1 teaspoon of medicine, he or she is to take 5 cc. The average household teaspoon holds between 2.5 and 7.8 cc or ml of liquid so it is not an accurate device for measuring medicine. Your pharmacy has inexpensive, accurate measuring devices to give liquid medicine. These devices come as droppers, medication cups, oral syringes, and spoonlike devices. When medicines come with their own calibrated droppers they should only be used with that specific medicine. The dropper is designed to measure that medicine accurately based on the medication's weight, viscosity, and specific gravity.

The liquid administration devices you purchase from the pharmacy can be reused after washing them with soap and water. The package label should indicate if the device is dishwasher safe. Injection syringes with the needle removed may also be used to administer liquid medicine. They often lose their calibration markings if placed in a dishwasher, so they must be carefully washed by hand. Oral medicine cups used by medical facilities are not dishwasher safe.

After you accurately measure and prepare the liquid medicine, it is necessary to consider how your child will react to this medicine. This helps you plan your approach to make the medicine experience a positive one.

Tablets and Capsules

In addition to liquids, oral medicines come in tablet and capsule forms. You must know whether your child can swallow either a tablet or a capsule before giving one. It is also a good idea to discuss with your physician which form of medicine would be best when the medicine is prescribed.

Some oral medications are manufactured only in tablet form. If your child is under five or unable to swallow a tablet, it must be

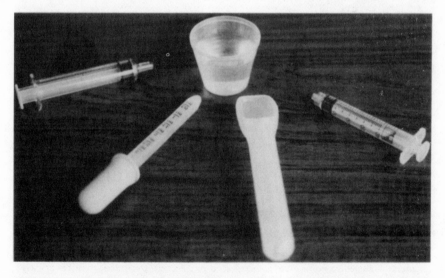

Devices used to measure liquid medications accurately. *From left to right:* oral syringe, dropper, medicine cup, spoonlike device, injection syringe without needle.

crushed. Either place the tablet inside a folded square of wax paper and crush it with a flat blunt object or use the bowl of one spoon and the back of another spoon to crush the tablet in between.

Certain tablets should not be crushed because this would adversely affect the medicine's action. For example, enteric-coated tablets, which are usually characterized by a shiny coating, should not be crushed because the coating is designed to prevent the drug from being destroyed in the stomach. Sustained-release tablets have ingredients embedded inside the tablet to achieve a gradual release of the drug in the body and should not be crushed. If you have questions about whether a specific tablet can be safely crushed, consult your pharmacist. Conversely, chewable tablets should be chewed or crushed but they should not be swallowed whole.

If your child is under five or is unable to swallow a capsule, it can be taken apart to extract the medicine inside. Just hold one end of the capsule in the upright position and gently pull the top section off. You will usually find a powdered form of the medicine inside the capsule. Some capsules contain colored round particles. These particles are a

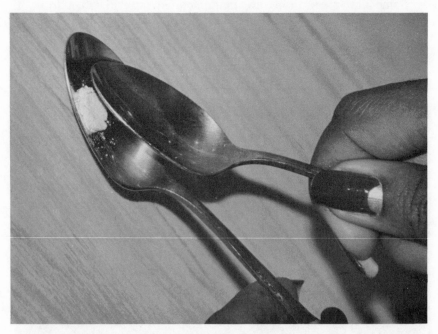

To make it easier to administer a tablet to a small child, the tablet may be crushed between two spoons. Place the tablet in the bowl of one spoon and press down with the back of the other spoon until the tablet is crushed. *(Sidney Cooper)*

sustained-release form of the medicine and can be removed from the capsule. Your child should be instructed not to chew the particles, which would destroy the protective coating.

Since tablets and the contents of capsules are usually bitter or unpleasant-tasting, it may be necessary to disguise the taste of the medicine. This can be done by mixing the medicine with food or fluid. You need to select this substance carefully and not place the medicine in an essential food like milk or orange juice, since the child may develop an aversion to the food or drink because the medication altered its taste. Some foods to consider using are jelly, honey, applesauce, ice cream, and fruit-flavored drink. The American Academy of Pediatrics recommends that honey not be used if the child is under twelve months of age because of evidence that honey, especially unprocessed honey, may contain a strain of botulism spore harmful to the infant.

If you are going to use a solid to mix with the medicine, place a small amount of food such as applesauce in a spoon. Carefully sprinkle

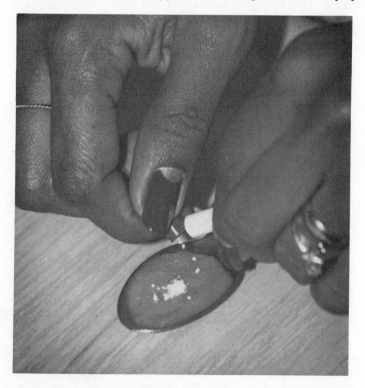

The contents of a capsule may be sprinkled onto a spoonful of applesauce before being given to a child. *(Sidney Cooper)*

the crushed tablet or contents of the capsule on the applesauce. Then place a very small amount of the applesauce over the medication, covering it completely. Prepare the mixture of applesauce and medicine in a small enough quantity so your child can take it all in one bite. This helps decrease contact between the medicine and your child's tongue and hopefully avoids the bad taste of the medicine. You may also mix a crushed tablet in a very small amount (about 15 cc or ½ ounce) of water or fruit-flavored drink. Never put the crushed tablet in a full glass of water or in a bottle of juice, because your child may not take all the fluid. Your child would not get the dosage prescribed, and it would be impossible to calculate how much medicine was received.

Positioning a Child to Receive Medicine by Mouth

No child should receive an oral medicine while lying down or flat on the back. This could cause choking and some of the medicine could get into the lungs. The child should be sitting up (at least at a 45-degree angle) or standing when given medicine by mouth.

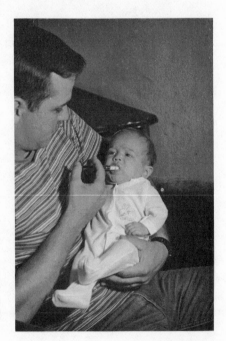

An infant receiving an oral medicine from a syringe. She is held with her head elevated 45 degrees; since she is so young, her hands and feet do not need to be restrained. *(Sidney Cooper)*

Infants Under Four Months

Position or hold the infant with the head elevated 45 degrees and hands and legs restrained as necessary. Until about four to six months of age the infant's tongue functions primarily for sucking, which causes spitting out of anything other than a nipple. You may have noticed this when you attempted to give solid food with a spoon. Liquid medicine should be placed in something that can be sucked from, such as a nipple, syringe, or dropper. The infant can suck the medicine directly from a dropper or syringe, and the medicine can be poured into an empty nipple for administration.

The sucking reflex is strong and can be elicited by placing the nipple, dropper, or syringe in the baby's mouth and lightly stroking the side of the cheek. Infants usually take medicine better if they are hungry.

The young infant's sense of taste is not as highly developed as that of an older child. Taste is best distinguished on the tip of the tongue, so if you place the medicine further back, it will usually not be as objectionable. However, if the medicine is an elixir (one that contains

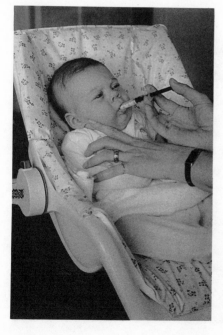

A young infant can be positioned in an infant seat to receive an oral medicine from a syringe. Notice that while the care provider administers the medicine with one hand, the child's hands are restrained and her head is stabilized by the other hand. *(Bil Paul)*

alcohol), give it slowly, since many infants seem to choke with this type of preparation.

If your infant sucks the medicine but seems hesitant or refuses to swallow, gently stroke downward on the throat. Do this right over the Adam's apple region of the throat.

If your infant chokes while taking the medicine, remove the medicine at once from the mouth and sit the child upright. Lift the baby's arms over her or his head and watch closely. If spitting up occurs, turn the child to the side and place the head downward to facilitate removal of fluid from the mouth. When the choking has stopped, reposition the infant and administer the remaining medicine.

Capsules must be taken apart and their contents removed and tablets must be crushed to give to a young infant. The medicine may be better accepted if it is mixed with a liquid and given in a nipple, syringe, or dropper. For the infant under three months, it is best to use apple juice or water if solids have not been introduced.

Infants Four Months to Twelve Months

The infant between three months and twelve months grasps and holds on to objects. Thus this child may attempt to grab the medicine

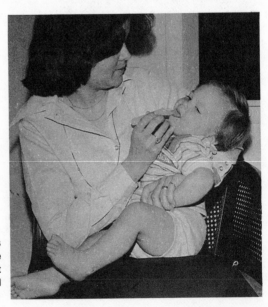

A nine-month-old infant receives oral medication from a spoonlike device. He is positioned so that both of his arms are restrained during administration.

administration device from you. To avoid this, position the child in an infant seat or propped up against pillows, and hold the baby's hands during administration.

Another method that works well with the older infant is to position the child in the following manner: Sit the child across your lap, facing the hand that is used to give the medicine. Put your infant's arm that is near your body along your side and under your arm. Grasp the child's free arm in the hand not giving the medicine. To control the child's head, place it against your shoulder. Use your free hand to give the medicine.

With the child over five or six months, the syringe, dropper, cup, or medicine spoon works better than the nipple. This is because the infant may pull the nipple from the mouth, thus spilling the medicine. Sometimes the medicine is readily sucked from the syringe or dropper and other times it is not. If your infant will not suck the medicine, you can place the syringe across the tongue, direct it toward the side of the mouth rather than the throat, and give it slowly. This serves two purposes. First, with the syringe across the tongue, the child will not be able to spit the medicine out. Second, directing the medicine downward and to the side of the mouth prevents choking or eliciting the cough reflex. You can also get the older infant to swallow by gently stroking downward on the throat.

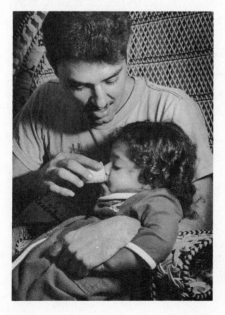

When giving a toddler medicine by mouth, restrain the hands and head to make administration easier. Notice that the care provider is using his shoulder to control the child's head movement while holding the child's free hand. *(Sidney Cooper)*

A child of this age still needs to have tablets crushed or capsules taken apart. The medicine can be administered in either a nonessential food, such as applesauce or jelly, or in 15 ccs, about ½ ounce, of fluid.

The Toddler (One to Three Years Old)

When you select a measuring device it is helpful to consider your child's personality and fears. For example, if injections are feared, it is best not to use a syringelike device for giving oral medicines, since your child may be afraid that an injection will be given into the mouth. The toddler usually takes liquid medicine best from a medicine spoon or cup, but your child may prefer a syringe or dropper. When a child does not cooperate with taking oral medicine, follow the administration procedure described for the older infant.

One of the biggest problems with children of this age is getting them to swallow what is in their mouths quickly, so that the bad taste will go away. They usually hold it in their mouths or attempt to spit it out. Sometimes you can get them to swallow quickly by offering sips of their favorite fluid in between taking the medicine; this is especially helpful if the medication tastes bad. Some parents have found that giving a child a popsicle or large piece of ice to suck on prior to taking the medicine helps to decrease the taste buds' acuity. Since toddlers feel secure with repetitive actions, tell the baby-sitter, nursery school teacher, or other caretaker the routines for taking medicines.

All tablets and capsules should be crushed or taken apart for this age group. The toddler may also need chewable tablets crushed if he or she is unable to comprehend instructions to chew the tablet.

The Preschooler (Three to Six Years)

This child usually cooperates and takes oral medicines. Medications can be taken from the cup or medicine spoon. Choices can be made by this age group, so if there is more than one medicine to take, the preschooler may wish to select the one to take first.

At about five to six years of age, the preschooler starts to lose teeth. Because of this chewable tablets can present a problem if a tooth is loose. The child could jar the tooth loose and swallow it. You may wish to crush chewable tablets prior to administration. Liquids and chewable or crushed tablets are the best choices for oral medicines, since most preschoolers have difficulty swallowing whole tablets or capsules.

The School-ager (Six to Twelve Years)

This child takes oral medications well and is usually able to swallow capsules and pills. If the school-ager cannot take tablets, your health care provider should be informed when medicine is required. This age child now understands time and is able to take responsibility. The school-ager may like to keep a chart or record by placing a star or sticker on a chart when the drug is taken.

If possible, it is best to plan the medicine schedule to avoid having to take any medication while in school. However, if it is necessary to take the medicine during school hours, the child may be able to take it or the teacher or school nurse may have to be responsible for the administration. Check with your child's school, since self-medication procedures may vary. Safety precautions should be followed so that other children do not have access to a potentially harmful medicine. If your school-ager must take medicine while in school, your child may benefit from discussing the illness and medicine during show-and-tell or sharing time. This is especially important if the child is on medication for a chronic illness, as it may help save face with peers. Children of this age group are very dependent upon their peer group for acceptance

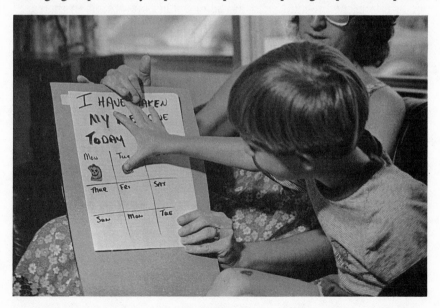

Children who cooperate with medicine administration can be rewarded by adding a sticker to their medicine chart. *(Sidney Cooper)*

and their sense of identity. If they view an illness such as diabetes as making them different, they may assume that their peers will not accept them. Some children then react by withdrawing from the group. The other children in the class can also benefit from this type of discussion by seeing that a child with an illness is not so different from themselves.

During the early years of school age, the child may still be losing baby teeth. Thus you will need to make sure a tooth is not dislodged if the child is taking a chewable tablet.

The Adolescent

The adolescent can usually administer and be responsible for medicines with proper instructions from the parent or the health care provider.

The adolescent needs to be knowledgeable about the medicine, including how the drug works, why it is necessary, and its unintended side effects. Many adolescents are tempted by peers and others to experiment with street drugs and alcohol. Certain prescription and nonprescription drugs interact unfavorably with alcohol and street drugs. For example, many of the street "speeds" contain phenylpropanolamine, which is present in many cold medicines. This may result in increased central nervous system (CNS) excitation, such as irritability and restlessness, not experienced with the normal dosage of cold medicines. Also, Flagyl (metronidazole), which is commonly prescribed for vaginal yeast infections, interacts with alcohol, resulting in an Antabuse type of reaction. Antabuse is a drug given to alcoholics to cause unfavorable symptoms to occur when alcohol is ingested. Metronidazole, like the drug Antabuse, interrupts alcohol decomposition by the liver, and toxic by-products build up in the bloodstream. As a result, when metronidazole and alcohol reach sufficient levels in the blood, symptoms appear ranging from flushing of the face, headache, nausea, vomiting, and shortness of breath, to unconsciousness, and if the intake of alcohol is high enough, it can lead to convulsion and death. Thus your child needs to be aware of this. Alcoholics who receive Antabuse are under close medical supervision.

If you suspect that your adolescent may be experimenting with drugs and you have trouble talking to your child about it, seek advice from a health care provider, since your teenager may discuss this problem more openly with a medical person than with you.

By Rectum

When your child is unable to tolerate food or fluids by mouth due to nausea or vomiting, rectal application of medication may be used. The suppository is the most common form.

A suppository contains medicine placed in a base of glycerin or lanolin that melts at body temperature. It should be stored in a cool place or in the refrigerator. Suppositories vary in shape and size but are usually cone-shaped. Use only suppositories designed for children. Do not divide an adult suppository, because the correct dosage cannot be guaranteed. Rectal suppositories are best absorbed when the rectum is empty of stool.

The instructions on the label indicate whether lubrication is needed prior to inserting the suppository into the child's rectum. Lubrication is accomplished by using a water-soluble gel, such as K-Y jelly, available at most pharmacies. If suppositories are prelubricated, this information appears on the instruction label.

Suppositories and enemas should not be given routinely to your child for laxative action. If on a rare occasion constipation occurs, a glycerin suppository may be used. It is best to consult your health care provider before giving it to your child. When suppositories or enemas are used on a daily or weekly basis, they interfere with bowel tone and can have long-term negative results. Consult your physician for an evaluation if constipation is a problem.

Enemas are not routinely used with children; therefore they are not discussed in this book. If an enema is prescribed for your child, be sure to obtain instructions on how to give it.

Preparing for the Administration of a Suppository

It is helpful to have everything ready prior to the suppository insertion so that you do not have to stop in the middle of the procedure. You will need the following items:

- the suppository
- a plastic glove or finger cot to protect your finger during insertion (available at a pharmacy)
- lubrication gel if necessary
- tissue or toilet paper to clean the rectal area following insertion
- another person if necessary to help hold the child during insertion

How to Give Rectal Medicine

The rectum is located in an area referred to as the perineum. The rectal opening is protected and controlled by the sphincter, a set of muscles that allow the child to have bowel control. The rectum is easily visualized in boys, between the buttocks and to the back of the scrotum. In girls the sphincter opening is between the buttocks and is the one of three openings located closest to the tailbone.

To insert a suppository, first position the child on her or his left side

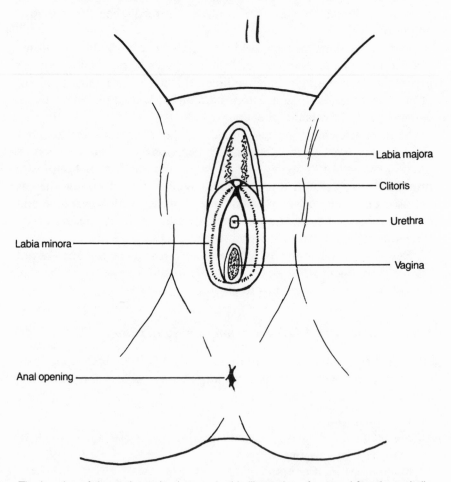

The location of the anal opening is seen in this illustration of external female genitalia.

and draw the child's knee to the chest. This is called a Sims' position. It is helpful to have a second person hold the child's legs, thereby preventing straightening of the legs and keeping the child correctly positioned. Separate the buttocks with the hand that is not inserting the suppository to visualize the rectal sphincter. Make sure you have the correct opening. Now carefully insert the suppository, pointed end first. Gently push the suppository into the rectal area past the sphincter with your gloved finger. The insertion of the suppository and your finger does not hurt the child if you use gentle pressure and do not force your finger when you feel resistance.

During the insertion of a suppository, if you meet with resistance it could be due to stool in the rectum. Gently place your gloved finger inside the child's rectum. If this is the problem, you will have stool on your finger upon removal. Stop the procedure and allow the child to have a bowel movement prior to the suppository insertion. The insertion of your finger into the rectum often stimulates a bowel movement. However, if you feel resistance and it is not stool or if your child appears to experience pain, do not force the suppository but consult your physician. If your child is having diarrhea, it is best not to use a suppository because it can stimulate the bowel further or it simply will not stay in the rectum long enough to be absorbed.

Immediately following the insertion of the suppository, your child is likely to feel the need to defecate and will probably try to accomplish this. By having a bowel movement at this time, the suppository will be expelled before the medicine can act. To prevent this from happening, have the child remain lying down and hold the buttocks together for five to ten minutes, until the urge to defecate has subsided.

If your child has a bowel movement within ten to thirty minutes following the insertion of a suppository, check the stool for the presence of the suppository. If the suppository was not given for laxative action and part of it is expelled, contact your health care provider before giving it again so the health care provider can evaluate the situation.

To the Infant (One to Twelve Months Old)

The infant does not understand explanations of suppository insertion, so the procedure is best done quickly and safely. Position the infant on his or her left side. Having a second person hold your infant in the

Sims' position prevents the child from turning over and will keep the legs in proper position. Give the infant a pacifier to suck on to create relaxation, distraction from the urge to defecate, and prevention of tightening of the rectal sphincter.

If your child is a full-term infant (not a premature infant) to a three-year-old, use your fourth or little finger to insert the suppository. Proceed as described in the giving of the rectal medicine. To help prevent the infant from expelling the suppository, pick up and hold the infant while

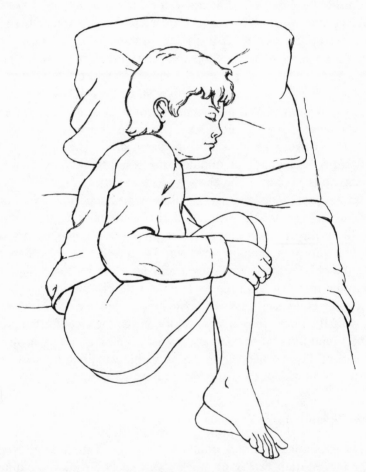

The insertion of a suppository is made easier when the child assumes the Sims' position. The legs are clasped to the body so they do not become straightened during the insertion.

also holding the buttocks together. Check the diaper every ten to fifteen minutes to see if the suppository has been expelled. Contact your health care provider if you have any questions.

To the Toddler (One to Three Years Old)

The toddler may not respond well to rectal medicines. Since the understanding of a child of this age is limited, explanations usually do not help. Thus it is best to give a very simple explanation while you are doing the procedure. If your child fights when you take a rectal temperature, the administration of a suppository will likely create the same behavior. Have an adult assist you if this is the situation, explaining that the suppository is medicine and not a punishment.

The suppository is given the same way as described in the section on giving rectal medicines to an infant. Instruct the toddler to pant like a puppy or pretend to be blowing out a candle during administration, to prevent tightening of the rectal sphincter muscles. If the younger toddler still uses a pacifier, have the child suck on it during the suppository insertion to increase relaxation. Following the insertion, the toddler's buttocks should be held together for five to ten minutes until the urge to defecate has subsided. Follow the same instructions for observing the expulsion of the suppository as described earlier.

To the Preschooler (Three to Six Years Old)

The preschooler usually is afraid of any rectal medicine, due to the fear of genital entry. Even if rectal medicine was given previously when the child was a toddler, you may see increased resistance now. You may need another adult to restrain the child. If he or she is cooperative, this age child may be able to place the arms under the knees and assist you in keeping the insertion position. The preschooler can pant like a puppy or pretend to blow out a candle to decrease the urge to defecate during the insertion. When the child is over three years of age, you may use your second or index finger to insert the suppository. Have the child remain lying down for five to ten minutes following the insertion of the suppository to prevent expulsion before the medicine can work in the rectum.

After the instillation of the suppository your child may benefit from having a doll to play with so feelings about this procedure can be acted out. Showing the child that the genitals are still intact following the procedure helps reduce the fear that the suppository may have harmed the body. These play opportunities and explanations help work out fears and frustrations the child may be unable to verbalize.

To the School-ager (Six to Twelve Years Old)

This age child can be cooperative because he or she can understand why a suppository must be given. But your child may become upset about the procedure and need a chance to express anxiety without ridicule. Allow your child privacy if crying occurs so the child does not lose face with siblings. Privacy also becomes important at about seven years of age, when most children develop a sense of modesty. This may occur earlier or later, depending on the child. These feelings should be respected.

Rectal medicine is given to a school-age child the same way it is to the child over three.

The Adolescent

If the adolescent needs a suppository it is given as described for younger children. Taking deep breaths during the insertion helps relax the rectal sphincter. The teenager should remain on his or her side for fifteen minutes to allow the suppository medicine to work.

The suppository can be self-administered. Be certain the adolescent knows the technique for insertion as described earlier.

To the Eye

The human eye is a sensitive and delicate organ. When applying medicine to the eye, follow a very clean technique to avoid the introduction of germs.

Medicine for the eye comes in two forms: liquid that is dispensed by dropper or squeeze bottle and ointment that is applied directly from the tube. Eye medicines are sterile (free from germs), and care must be taken not to contaminate them, which introduces germs, or injure the eye during the administration of the medicine.

Eyedrops usually come in small bottles, since very small amounts are required for treatment of the eye. The medicine is dispensed from a dropper or directly from a plastic bottle with a special tip for administration. The end of the dropper or plastic-tipped bottle should never touch the eye, the eyelashes, or the hands of the individual administering the medication. The medicine may be prescribed for one or both eyes, depending on the condition. Administer only the amount of medicine prescribed, because altering the amount of drops could be harmful to the eye. Store liquid eye medicines at room temperature, because cold solutions are irritating to the eye and cause the child to blink.

Eye ointments are dispensed in a tube. Store them at room temperature unless instructed otherwise. If you have previously used the ointment from this tube, before using it again, squeeze out a small amount of the medicine onto a clean tissue without touching the tube tip to the tissue. Discard the medicine on the tissue. This clears the tube and removes medicine that may have become contaminated during the previous instillation or storage.

How to Give Eye Medicine

Position the child flat on the back with a pillow under the neck and elevating the shoulders. When the child's head is lower than the body, gravity helps spread the medicine over the cornea.

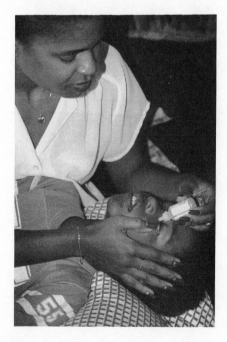

To administer eye medicine to a child, begin with the child lying down, with the neck hyperextended over a pillow. The child's eyes should be closed. Rest the hand that administers the medicine on the child's forehead. Use the other hand to retract the lower lid, and instill the prescribed number of drops. *(Sidney Cooper)*

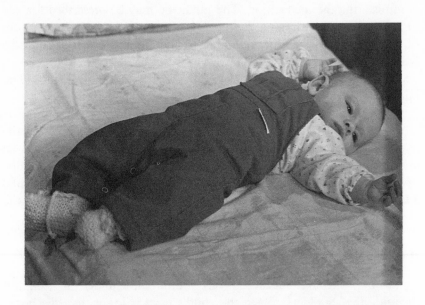

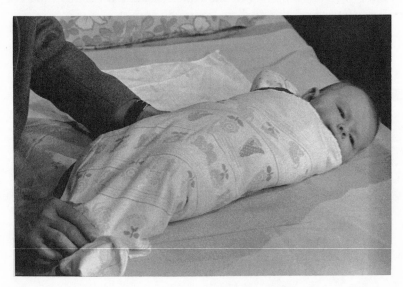

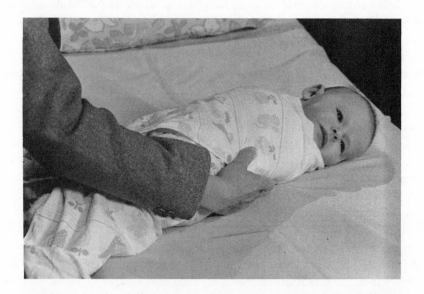

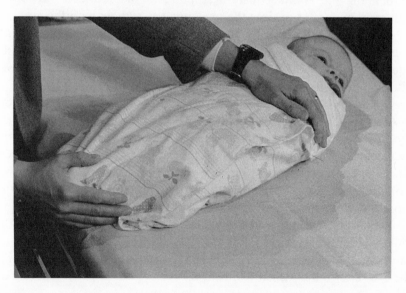

A four-step procedure secures an infant in a mummy restraint. (1) Lay the child in the upper-middle portion of a large blanket. The edge of the blanket should touch the child's neck. (2) Place the child's right arm flat against his right side and wrap the blanket over the child's body, securing the right arm. (3) Place the child's left arm against the body and wrap the blanket over the body to secure the left arm. (4) Fold the lower end of the blanket onto the child's chest. In a mummy restraint, the arms, legs, hands, and feet are secured. *(Roy Ramsey)*

It is natural for your child to fear having anything placed in the eye. It is an especially frightening experience to see a dropper coming toward the eye. Your child may react by closing the eye so tightly that it seems it will never open. It works best to instruct your child to close his or her eyes. This helps lessen fears and prevents the child from looking at the dropper. Rest the hand that is going to be used to give the medicine on the child's forehead. This helps to stabilize the hand and prevents you from inadvertently pushing the dropper or tube into the child's eye. Using the other hand, gently retract the lower lid by carefully applying pressure downward on the skin directly below the eye. Since the eye area is sensitive, take care when doing this. When the lid is retracted, you will note that a saclike area has been formed by the inner wall of the lid and the eye. With a liquid eye medicine, place the specified number of drops in the appropriate eye, taking care not to touch the eye or any adjacent structures with the end of the dropper. Do not place the drop onto the colored portion of the eye, because this can cause an uncomfortable sensation, stimulating the child to tear or blink. Crying or blinking prevents adequate absorption of the medicine because it reduces the amount of time the medicine has contact with the eye.

Have the child remain in this hyperextended position for at least five minutes with the eyes closed to ensure that the medicine has adequate contact with the eye. Prevent the child from rubbing the eyes after the drops have been administered.

For an ointment, position your child in the same manner as for the instillation of eyedrops. Retract the lower lid the same way and squeeze the tube gently; this will cause a small line of ointment to fall into the saclike area of the lid. Do not touch the end of the tube to the eye area. To stop the ointment flow, rotate the tube with a twisting motion and stop squeezing the tube. Return the lower lid to its normal position and have the child remain lying down with the eyes closed. The child's vision will be blurred by the instillation of the ointment. When the child opens the eyes, explain that this blurring will pass in several minutes; this will help reduce the fear. Prevent the child from rubbing the eyes after the ointment is instilled.

To an Infant (One to Twelve Months Old)

Have the infant lie on a flat surface for the instillation of eyedrops or ointment. Mummy-restrain the child or have another adult restrain the child's arms and legs so you can focus on giving the medicine.

Proceed as described. It may be difficult to retract just the lower lid of the infant, because the area is so small. You can open the eyelids by gently pushing the lids open and exposing the eye. With the thumb on the upper lid and the index finger on the lower lid, use gentle pressure in opposite directions to open the eye of an infant. Do not put pressure on the eyeball itself. Remember that the eye area is sensitive. Place the drops or ointment along the lower lid area, avoiding the colored part of the eye.

Hold the infant horizontally for two to five minutes following administration. This provides comfort and allows the medicine to remain in contact with the eye longer.

To a Toddler (One to Three Years)

The toddler is usually frightened by eye medicines. Sometimes it helps to have your child watch you close your own eyes and pull down on your lower lid and then have the child copy your action. The child can see that this does not hurt. With this age group it is best to have another adult help give the medicine. One adult will hold the child,

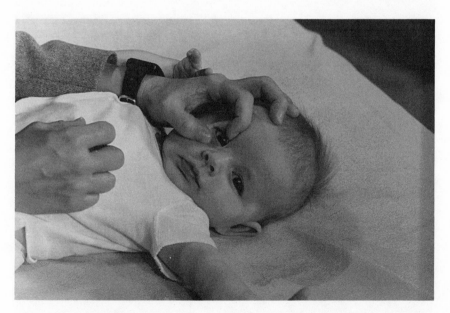

To open an infant's eye to administer eye medication: with the thumb on the lower lid and the index finger on the upper lid, use gentle pressure in opposite directions to open the eyelid of an infant. Do not put pressure on the eyeball itself. *(Roy Ramsey)*

stabilizing the head, and the other adult can concentrate on giving the medicine. If you find yourself alone and if the child is under two, a mummy restraint may be used. Having another adult assist you is beneficial in case the child cooperates in the beginning but becomes upset and later fights the procedure. Position and give the drops or ointment as described.

To a Preschooler (Three to Six Years)

This age group responds to simple directions and explanations of the procedure, such as, "Lie down and close your eyes." This instruction is best given just prior to the administration of the eyedrops. The preschooler may also benefit from closing the eyes and pulling down the lower lid to learn that this does not hurt. Restrain the child as necessary, position her or him, and give the medicine as described.

It may be helpful for the child to see and play with an old dropper, which can be used to give the eye medicine to dolls or stuffed toys. The use of play helps the child vent feelings and frustrations.

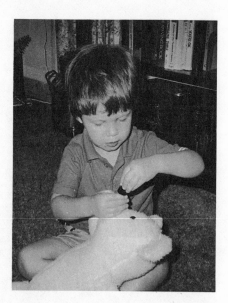

Allowing a preschooler to play with an old dropper and give his stuffed bear nose-drops helps to lessen any fear or anxiety the child may harbor about receiving nosedrops. *(Sidney Cooper)*

To a School-ager or an Adolescent

Children this age usually cooperate well with eye medicine administration. Instill as described.

For the Ear

Ear medicine comes in liquid form and is administered by dropper. The health care provider prescribes the number of drops to be placed in a particular ear.

The eardrops should be kept at room temperature, since cold drops may cause pain when instilled. If the ear is draining, always check with your physician before giving this medicine to your child. A draining ear may indicate that the eardrum has ruptured; when this is so, the solution could enter the inner ear. Only freshly prescribed medicine should be placed in a draining ear. In addition, never irrigate an ear, draining or not, with a myringotomy tube. Myringotomy tubes (P.E. tubes) are very tiny tubes that are surgically placed in a child's ears as a method for treating persistent, chronic ear infections. If tubes are in place in the eardum, you could dislodge them or introduce infection into the inner ear by irrigating them.

How to Give Ear Medicine

Place the child on his or her side with the affected ear exposed. If the eardrops are given for an external otitis or a middle ear infection, the child may experience pain upon positioning of the ear for the drops. Should this be the case, adequately restrain and proceed quickly, then provide comfort following the instillation. The position of the ear for instillation depends on the child's age (see appropriate section for correct positioning). When administering the drops, take care to direct them so they fall along the wall of the ear canal. This prevents the drops from directly hitting the eardrum, which can produce nausea or vomiting. Massage the exterior ear gently following the instillation to ease the entry of the drops into the canal. Have the child remain lying in the position used to instill the medicine so the drops have a chance to reach the eardrum.

To an Infant (One to Twelve Months Old)

The infant under six to nine months of age can be held on your lap or placed on a flat surface with the affected ear exposed. If your infant does not cooperate by lying still, have someone assist you. To instill the drops, gently pull the earlobe downward and backward. This helps to straighten and separate the walls of the ear canal and permits better instillation. Proceed with the instillation of drops as described. After the instillation, hold your infant in your arms with the affected ear upright for a few minutes to allow the eardrops to reach the eardrum. Comfort the child as necessary.

To a Toddler (One to Three Years Old)

Most toddlers cooperate with the instillation of eardrops. Administer the eardrops as described for the infant. Until the child is three years of age, pull the earlobe downward and back for the instillation of eardrops.

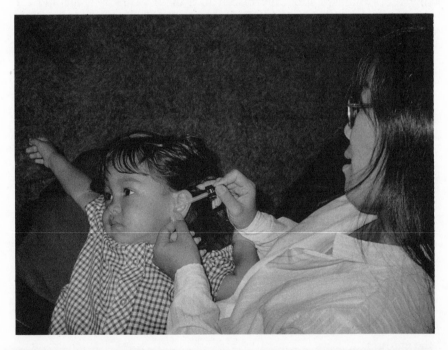

To administer eardrops to a child under three, the earlobe is gently pulled down and back.

To a Preschooler (Three to Six Years Old)

Eardrops are given as described for younger children. However, because this child has grown, the angle of the ear canal has changed. Therefore, with a child over three years old, the upper portion of the outer ear is gently pulled upward and back. This age child can lessen fears by playing with a dropper and a doll.

To a School-ager and an Adolescent

The ear is positioned by gently pulling the outer portion upward and back to separate the walls of the ear canal. Give the medicine as described on page 55.

By the Nose

Medicine is placed in the nose to ease breathing or to clean the nasal area. Because the instillation of nosedrops may produce a sensation of tickling, an unpleasant taste in the mouth, or difficulty in breathing,

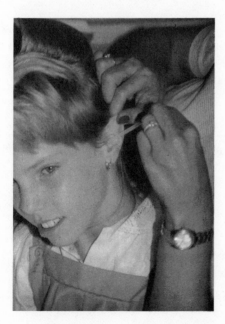

Gently pull the outer portion of the ear upward and back to separate the walls of the ear canal when giving eardrops to an adolescent.

your child may refuse to cooperate. To prevent injury during the instillation of nosedrops, it is necessary to restrain the young child adequately and to gain the cooperation of the older child.

How to Give Nosedrops

The child should be positioned with the head slightly lower than the rest of the body. Have the child lie down and place a pillow under the shoulders to lower the head. Your child's face should be looking directly at you and should be kept still during administration of the drops. You may need to mummy restrain or have another adult hold the child.

Medicine for the nose comes in liquid form; only drops labeled for instillation into the nose should be used. The health care provider will prescribe the exact number of drops to be placed in each nostril. After you place the correct number of drops in the nostrils, keep the child on her or his back with the head lower than the body to allow gravity to facilitate the action of the drops. When giving nosedrops, observe for choking, because the dripping of the medicine down the back of the throat can sometimes create a choking sensation. If choking or vomiting occurs, immediately turn the child to the side, keeping the head lower than the body, until the choking stops.

To an Infant (One to Twelve Months)

An infant up to six or nine months of age can be placed on your lap during the administration of nosedrops, with your knees lowered to position the head properly. The infant may also be positioned with the body on a pillow and the head lower. Be sure to use a relatively flat pillow to avoid over-hyperextension of the neck. Give the nosedrops as described. Have a bulb syringe ready for suctioning and use it if the infant's nostrils become filled with mucus. (See Appendix 3 for how to suction an infant's nose.) Hold and comfort the infant following the procedure.

To a Toddler (One to Three Years)

Most toddlers do not like nosedrops because of the choking and tickling sensation they may produce. Adequately restrain the child and closely observe him or her for signs of choking. A bulb syringe works well for the removal of excess mucus with this age group. Follow the instruction above on giving nosedrops.

To a Preschooler (Three to Six Years Old)

Give nosedrops as described on page 58 and observe the child for signs of choking. Again, the child can vent frustrations and fears through play with a dropper and doll.

To a School-ager and an Adolescent

This age child can be positioned across the parent's lap or positioned with a pillow under the neck to lower the head slightly for the administration of nosedrops. The older child may be able to self-administer nosedrops without the assistance of an adult. The child should lie down and place a pillow under the neck to lower the head and give the nosedrops as described on page 58.

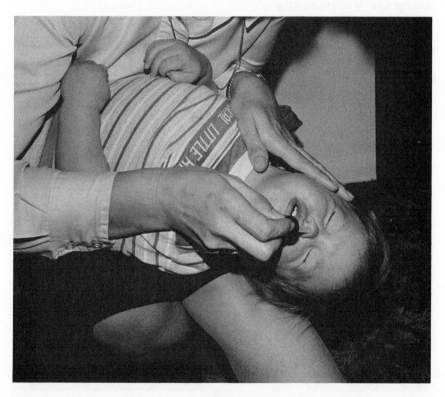

The head of a nine-month-old infant is placed lower than his body to receive nosedrops.

Nebulizer

A hand-held nebulizer is a piece of equipment that is sometimes used with bronchodilator medicine for the child who has asthma. The nebulizer should only be used for the relief of asthma as prescribed by a physician. When a bronchodilator is indicated, it is strictly for relief of symptoms; it is not a cure for asthma. Overuse of the bronchodilator may increase unintended effects. If a nebulizer is prescribed for your child, have the health care provider demonstrate how to use it correctly.

For the Skin and Hair

Applying medicine to the skin is one of the most common ways of treating a child at home. Medicated skin treatments contain a variety of substances to treat a number of conditions. These include shampoos for such problems as eczema and head lice; cleaning agents; ointments, lotions, and creams for antisepsis, itching, and rashes; and baths to treat allergies or skin poisonings.

Most topical (skin) products come with specific instructions either from the manufacturer or the health care provider. These must be read

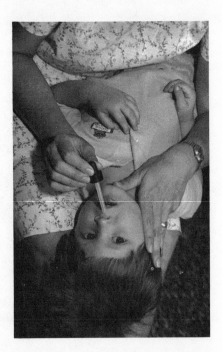

A two-year-old lies with his neck hyper-extended over his mother's knees to receive nosedrops. *(Sidney Cooper)*

carefully and adhered to as closely as possible. People tend to increase the amount of medicine applied or to apply it more frequently than directed. This does not speed healing but, instead, may result in undesired effects from the treatment.

Inspect the skin area involved on your child before and after the application of the medicine. Significant changes can occur within several hours, so close observation is needed to prevent the spread of infection. New pink tissue and drying indicate that the skin is healing. Redness and swelling, change in color of any drainage from clear to cloudy and thick, foul odor, or increased heat all indicate the presence of infection. If this occurs, notify your health care provider, because your child may need a change in treatment.

How to Use a Medicated Shampoo

With a noncontagious scalp problem such as eczema, shampoo the child's hair as directed on the product label. If your child's hair is being treated with a medicated shampoo for a contagious problem, such as head lice, refer to Chapter 12 for directions.

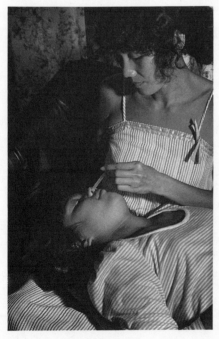

The neck of an adolescent is hyperextended over a pillow placed on her mother's lap to receive nosedrops. *(Sidney Cooper)*

When using a medicated shampoo, there are some general principles to consider. Carefully examine the scalp area before and after shampooing to note any changes in the scalp condition. Shampooing the hair while bathing in a tub is not recommended, because the medicated shampoo may irritate the skin of the body, especially in the genital region. It is better to use a bathroom or kitchen sink. Rinsing the hair is best accomplished by using a container such as a plastic cup or glass to pour water over the head. This prevents the rinse water from entering the child's eyes. A sink spray hose can also be used for this purpose. Take care to avoid getting rinse water into the child's ears.

Likewise, nonprescription skin products such as medicated shampoos are to be used according to manufacturer's directions. Care should be taken to avoid contact of medicated shampoos with your child's eyes. The chemicals contained in the shampoo can be very irritating.

How to Apply Topical Medicines to the Skin

When applying a topical agent to an intact, noncontagious skin condition, a clean process is used. Gloves may be used to apply lotions or creams, or you may use your clean hands. Disposable plastic gloves are available at your pharmacy. Clean applicators such as wooden tongue blades or cotton-tipped swabs can be used to apply creams and ointments. A thin coat of medicine is sufficient unless otherwise directed. If the ointment stings or burns, the child may not cooperate and another person is needed to hold the child during the application. Some lotions and creams stain clothes and other material; be sure to read the label and take appropriate precautions.

A cut or break in the skin is considered an open wound. The most common childhood injuries you will encounter are skinned areas, cuts, and insect bites. Restrain the child as necessary and seek another adult to help you as needed when cleaning and applying medicine to the skin.

The wound needs to be cleaned before the application of any antiseptic. You can use a gauze pad, cotton-tipped applicator, or clean white washcloth with an antiseptic cleaning agent. (Use a clean washcloth to clean only very superficial wounds.) Start at the center of the wound and clean outward. This prevents germs on the outer edge of the wound from being introduced to the center. Discard the disposable cleaning applicator after one use.

Use another applicator to apply creams gently in the center first, and another to cover the outer edges. If you are uncertain about how to clean the wound or if you feel the wound needs medical attention, consult your health care provider.

If the wound needs a bandage, make sure the gauze portion completely covers the open area of the wound. Bandages come in various sizes and have such properties as being flexible and permeable, allowing air to pass through the sticky portion. Make sure the area to which the tape is applied is dry so it adheres. Use tape sparingly, because some children are allergic to tape and skin can break down under tape. The skin under the tape may appear reddened or the skin tissue may actually be broken and open.

To an Infant (One to Twelve Months Old)

Apply skin medicine as described. Since the infant cannot respond to verbal instructions not to scratch or rub skin lesions if they itch, you may need to mitten the hands or use specially designed gowns and shirts that have built-in coverings for the hands. Keep the infant's nails short and clean to prevent the introduction of germs into the lesion. As soon as your infant can put things into her or his mouth, you will need to take special care if the medicine is applied to the hands or feet to make sure the child cannot get these into the mouth.

Use adhesive tape sparingly on an infant, since many infants under six months old are sensitive to it. Also read the labels on all nonprescription creams and lotions to make sure they are safe to use with infants. Infants absorb topical agents more readily from their skin than older children do.

To a Toddler (One to Three Years Old)

The toddler may become upset over a skin abrasion or cut because seeing blood is scary. Encourage cooperation by distracting attention from the wound. If itching is a problem with a rash or an open wound, have the child wear mittens as necessary, especially when sleeping. If itching remains a problem, contact your health care provider so something can be prescribed. Keep the child's nails short and clean.

To a Preschooler (Three to Six Years Old)

The preschooler becomes frightened by rashes, abrasions, and cuts. Since he or she often views the skin as a container that holds blood and other body parts in, the child may worry that his or her insides will fall out when there is a break in the skin. Reassure your child that this will not happen. Using plastic adhesive strips and wound dressings helps alleviate fears; in fact, the child may become more upset when the dressings are removed.

This age child usually follows verbal instructions not to scratch a rash or wound, especially if distracted with things to do. During naps and at night cover the hands with mittens as necessary. To prevent the introduction of secondary infections, keep the nails short and clean. If itching is a problem, contact your health care provider.

To a School-ager (Six to Twelve Years Old)

This child understands the reason and instructions for applying creams and lotions. Sometimes less pain and anxiety are experienced by the child if he or she is allowed to remove the plastic adhesive strips or dressings on an open wound.

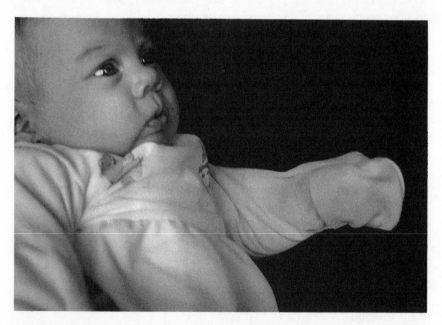

When infants suffer from a rash they are likely to scratch or rub, their hands can be covered by specially designed gowns and shirts until the skin heals. *(Bil Paul)*

If the school-ager has a skin ailment in which itching is a problem, hands should be covered with mittens at night. Medication may be needed for the itching. Keep the nails short and clean.

To an Adolescent

The adolescent can be responsible for wound care. It is helpful, however, to check the wound occasionally to ensure that proper care has been taken and there is no infection.

Vaginal Medicines

Infants, toddlers, preschoolers, and school-agers rarely need vaginal medications. If your daughter needs this type of medicine, have your health care provider give you detailed instructions on how to instill the drug.

The vagina is located between the urethra and the anal opening. In the young adolescent who has not used tampons or had a pelvic exam, this area may seem small; however, it will expand to allow the insertion of an applicator.

Since the vaginal area is a sexual organ, it is important for both you and your daughter to be in touch with your feelings. Your daughter may feel bad or unclean if a vaginal infection is present. Your reactions and feelings can be transmitted to your daughter. If you have any negative feelings about vaginal infections, you can make the child feel that something is wrong. Openness and a matter-of-fact attitude allow discussion of these feelings and assist relegating the vaginal medicine to its proper place as a treatment without negative connotations.

To an Adolescent

If you are to apply the medicine for your daughter, you will need good visualization because of the location of the vaginal opening and also to minimize discomfort. Have your daughter lie on her back with her knees flexed and spread apart. Locate the vaginal entrance and gently insert the medicine, pushing the applicator toward the child's spine. After the medication is inserted, have the adolescent remain lying down for several minutes. If your daughter stands up immediately, the medicine will leak out. Since a small amount of the medicine may leak out during the day, a small minipad or panty liner will prevent the medicine from soiling her undergarments. This liner should be changed frequently, as should the undergarments. If the medicine is only prescribed once a day, insert it before bedtime. The vaginal applicator needs to be washed in hot soapy water following each application. Only use the applicator for one person to reduce the spread of infection.

If your daughter is old enough to instill the vaginal medicine herself, teach the procedure as described. A hand-held mirror enables better visualization of the perineal area, or the adolescent may be able to feel the opening. If you are uncomfortable teaching your daughter, ask the doctor or nurse to give the instructions.

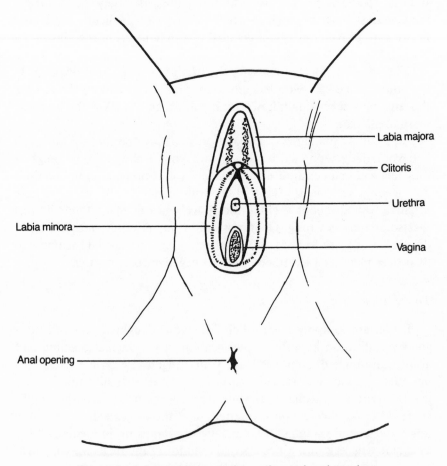

The vagina is located between the urethra and anal openings.

To further aid in the healing of vaginal infections it is best not to use deodorant tampons, since the medication and the deodorant chemical could react and further irritate the perineum. Also it is recommended that your daughter wear underpants that have a cotton crotch, since cotton allows for better air flow than do synthetic fabrics.

PART TWO

Immunizations

CHAPTER 5

Immunizations

Immunizations are one group of medicines all of you should make sure your child receives. Most of us no longer remember the epidemics, deaths, and permanent disabilities resulting from diseases that have now been greatly reduced by immunizations. The disease smallpox has even been totally eradicated, so that immunization against this disease is no longer required.

Although immunizations themselves are not totally without risk, the incidence of side effects is clearly and substantially less than the risk of permanent disability from the corresponding diseases. Precautions are taken in order to decrease the incidence of side effects. Immunizations are not given to someone who has an illness with a high fever, but a slight cold is not a contraindication. Someone who is receiving antibiotics, who is on medicines that suppress the immune system, who is pregnant, or who has chronic blood disease or cancer will not receive immunizations. In addition, measles-mumps-rubella vaccine is usually not given to someone with an allergy to eggs, chickens, ducks, or the antibiotic neomycin, since small amounts of these substances may be present in the vaccine. Be sure to inform your health care provider prior to immunization if your child has any special health conditions, allergies, or is taking any medicines.

Lack of adequate immunization in some communities and among certain age groups has allowed the incidence of communicable diseases to rise, so you need to be diligent in ensuring that your child is fully immunized. Many school systems now require proof of immunization, such as a card with dates from your doctor's office or health department.

A sample immunization record you can keep is shown here. Parents who are philosophically or religiously opposed to immunization need to sign a statement concerning this, and their children will be excluded from school if an outbreak of a communicable disease occurs.

Many parents have their children's immunizations administered during well-child visits to their health care provider. Most county health departments also administer immunizations at regularly scheduled clinics, either free or for a nominal charge. If you did not have your child immunized in infancy, you can still do so later. The schedule varies from that used in infancy (see Table 1) due to a more mature immune system. If your child received some immunizations in infancy but not a complete series, bring the list of those received to your health care provider, since there is no need to begin the whole series over again.

How Immunizations Work

The organisms that cause communicable diseases make protein substances known as *antigens*. They induce our body's immune system to produce *antibodies* to fight the diseases. An antibody is specific for a certain antigen, preventing only one disease. If the body is exposed by immunization to a weakened form of a communicable disease or to a toxin produced by the disease, it produces antibodies without actually suffering from a complete case of the disease. The body is then immune to that disease. This is the basis upon which immunization achieves its effect. Immunizations are effective in inducing the body to produce antibodies in 90 to 95 percent of all persons immunized.

Several types of substances can be used to produce an antibody:

Toxoid—a toxin (harmful substance) that is produced by the disease organism and is treated by heat or chemical. The treatment weakens the toxin but the body recognizes it as harmful and produces corresponding antibodies. Diphtheria and tetanus immunizations are examples of toxoids.

Vaccine—a preparation of dead or live organisms that are weakened to prevent disease occurrence but are capable of causing the body to produce antibodies against the disease. The immunization for pertussis, commonly known as whooping cough, is a vaccine of dead pertussis organisms, while oral polio, measles, mumps, and rubella vaccines contain live viruses.

Antitoxins and immune serum globulins—antibodies from people or animals who have been exposed to certain diseases. These are used in epidemics to produce short-term, nonpermanent protection from diseases.

Toxoids, vaccines, and the diseases themselves produce *active im-*

SUGGESTED
IMMUNIZATION SCHEDULE
for
SCHOOL CHILDREN AND ADULTS
NOT PREVIOUSLY IMMUNIZED

TETANUS-DIPHTHERIA (Td)

Two injections 2 months apart with a third injection six months to one year after the second; thereafter, a booster each 10 yrs.

POLIO

(not routinely recommended for persons above 18 years of age)

Two doses (taken by mouth) 2 months apart followed by a third dose 6 months to one year later.

MEASLES/MUMPS/RUBELLA (M-M-R)

(not routinely recommended for post-pubertal females)

One dose of this vaccine will provide protection against all three diseases.

DSHS 13-255 (X) Rev. 5-77

IMMUNIZATION
RECORD

| (Last Name) | (First) | (M.I.) |

| (Birthdate) | (Sex) |

| (Street or R.F.D.) |

| (City or Town) | (State) | (Zip) |

| (Physician, Clinic, or Health Department) |

| (Telephone Number) |

SUGGESTED IMMUNIZATION SCHEDULE
(for infants and children)

Ages	Vaccines
2 Months	1st DTP & 1st Polio
4 Months	2nd DTP & 2nd Polio
6 Months	3rd DTP & 3rd Polio*
18 Months	4th DTP & 4th Polio
4-6 Years	5th DTP & 5th Polio
15 Months	Measles, Mumps, & Rubella (M—M—R)

BOOSTER (Td)

Needed at 14-16 years of age and every 10 years thereafter	Td (Adult Type) Tetanus and diphtheria

*Third Polio dose optional

Children, whether on the above schedule or not, need 3 DTP and 2 POLIO in the first year; a 4th DTP & 3rd POLIO 12 months later; with boosters at 4-6 years; and M-M-R vaccine at 15 months or after.

DATES VACCINES ADMINISTERED

DTP	Polio	Td
1)	1)	
2)	2)	
3)	3)	
4)	4)	
5)	5)	
Measles	Mumps	Rubella

Notes:

TUBERCULIN SKIN TEST

Type of Test			
Date Given			
Date Read			
Reaction			

A sample immunization record, obtainable from your child's doctor or from the health department. You can record all immunizations your child receives. *(From State of Washington, Department of Social and Health Services, Immunization Program.)*

munity. This means that the person's body produces antibodies to counteract the disease. Such immunity is usually long-term, often lasting for life.

Antitoxins, immune serum globulin, and immunity acquired from the mother when the baby is in the uterus or drinking breast milk produce *passive immunity.* This immunity is temporary, generally lasting no more than a few months.

Recommended Immunizations

Diphtheria and Tetanus Toxoids and Pertussis Vaccine (DTP)

This immunization provides immunity to diphtheria, tetanus, often called lockjaw, and pertussis, all of which are serious diseases that can lead to death. Diphtheria is a bacterium that causes a severe sore throat, cough, fever, and respiratory infection, leading to death in half of the untreated cases. Tetanus is caused by an organism commonly found in soil, dust, and animal feces. The organism usually enters the body

Table 1   Immunization Schedule for Normal Infants and Children

Age	Immunizations	Method of Administration
2 mo	Diphtheria-tetanus-pertussis (DTP) TOPV (Polio)	Into muscle of thigh By mouth
4 mo	DTP TOPV	Into muscle of thigh By mouth
6 mo	DTP TOPV*	Into muscle of thigh By mouth
12 mo	TB test	Under skin of forearm
15 mo	Measles-mumps-rubella (MMR)	Into upper outer arm
18 mo	DTP TOPV	Into muscle of arm or thigh By mouth
24 mo	Haemophilus influenzae type B	Into upper outer arm
4–6 yrs	DTP TOPV	Into muscle of arm or thigh By mouth
14–16 yrs & every 10 yrs after	Tetanus-diphtheria (TD)	Into muscle of arm

* Optional dose.

Note: This schedule will vary for a child not immunized in early infancy.

Adapted from *Report of the Committee on Infectious Diseases,* 19th edition, "Redbook," 1982, p. 7.

through a wound and causes muscular tension, spasm, body stiffening, pain, and clenched jaws ("lockjaw"). Tetanus leads to death for half of the children and adults who contract the disease. The pertussis bacillus also causes a respiratory infection and a cough with a characteristic whoop. Pertussis is often a mild disease in children over one year and in adults. However, when infants are infected, it is much more serious and can even lead to death.

The DTP immunization is injected into a muscle by needle, usually into the thigh of infants and the upper arm of older children. It is administered at two, four, six, eighteen months, and between four to six years (see Table 1). A booster dose of diphtheria and tetanus is then needed every ten years. For wounds acquired five years or more after the last tetanus injection, a reimmunization should be given. More frequent injection could increase the chance of side effects. Pertussis vaccine is not given after seven years of age, since the disease does not occur often in older children or adults and the side effects of the immunization increase with age.

Unintended Effects

Common unintended effects of the DTP injection include redness, tenderness, swelling, or a lump at the injection site; low-grade fever (99°–102° F); fussiness, sleepiness, or changes in appetite. These are all temporary, usually occurring during the first and second days after immunization. A small pea-size lump may remain at the injection site for several months but gradually disappears. Acetaminophen is often given for a day or two following injection to alleviate the fever and tenderness (see discussion of this medicine in Chapter 6). A cool washcloth applied over the site can also decrease some of the tenderness.

Occasionally there are more severe reactions to the pertussis part of DTP (in 1 child in over 100,000 immunized). These include high fever (over 105° F), screaming, excessive sleepiness, and seizures. Should any of these side effects occur in your child, notify your health care provider immediately. Future doses of pertussis vaccine will likely be withheld so that your child receives only diphtheria and tetanus toxoids. Children with neurologic illness such as uncontrolled seizures are more likely to have a reaction to pertussis vaccine. Inform your health care provider prior to immunization if your child has a neurologic problem so that pertussis vaccine can be avoided if appropriate.

Trivalent Oral Polio Vaccine (TOPV or Polio)

Polio is caused by one of three related viruses that attack the spinal cord and brain stem, causing weakness, paralysis, breathing difficulty, and in 10 percent of cases, death.

The polio vaccine taken by mouth produces immunity to all three types of polio and is generally given on the same schedule as DTP: two, four, six, eighteen months, and four to six years (see Table 1). The third dose, usually given at about six months, is optional and so is not always given. Boosters after the dose at four to six years are not usually required.

Unintended Effects

Reactions to polio vaccine are extremely rare. One person in every three to four million immunized may actually contract polio and its resultant paralysis. Since the polio vaccine is a live virus that travels through, multiplies in, and is excreted from the intestinal tract, you as parents should be cautious in disposing of your infant's dirty diapers for the week or two following immunization, and inform other caretakers to do likewise. Wash your hands well after each diaper change, especially if you or other caretakers have not received full polio immunization.

Measles, Mumps, and Rubella Vaccines (MMR)

The diseases measles, mumps, and rubella are dangerous because of their associated problems. Measles (red "hard" measles) is characterized by fever, sore throat, white spots in the mouth, and a rash that begins on the face and travels downward to the rest of the body. In one person out of every three thousand with the disease, measles leads to encephalitis, a brain inflammation that can cause permanent damage. Mumps is caused by a virus that most commonly infects the salivary glands in the mouth but can also affect other organs such as the brain, ears, and the testicles or ovaries, sometimes leading to sterility. Rubella, or German measles, is caused by a virus that creates a rash and few other serious symptoms. The most serious complication of rubella occurs when it is contracted by a woman in the first three months of pregnancy; her child can be born with a variety of birth defects, such as vision loss, hearing impairment, mental retardation, and heart defects.

There has been a substantial number of cases of measles and rubella among United States college students in recent years. These have occurred because some college students are not adequately immunized for these diseases and because the diseases are easily transmitted in the close living quarters of college. If your daughter or son is in college or is college-bound, verify her or his health records to be certain an MMR was administered to the child after one year of age. It is wise to provide a copy of immunizations and dates received for your son or daughter who is heading away from home for work or college.

The MMR vaccine produces immunity to measles, mumps, and rubella. It is injected into fat tissue, usually in the upper outer arm, and is given at fifteen months of age. One injection appears to produce lifelong immunity. However, in case of an epidemic of measles, infants above six months may be immunized but the immunization is repeated at about fifteen months, since the immature immune system of the younger infant does not respond as reliably to the vaccine. In past years it was common to give the measles vaccine at an earlier age. If your child was immunized before one year, there may not have been an adequate immune response and reimmunization is needed. Some children received only one or two of the vaccines separately or received a killed rather than live virus measles vaccine (which was used from 1963–68). These persons should be immunized now by the presently available MMR vaccine.

Unintended Effects

Low-grade fever (up to 102° F) one to two weeks after immunization, a measleslike noncontagious rash in five to ten days, temporary joint pain, and redness at the injection site are occasional and harmless side effects of the MMR vaccines.

The MMR is not recommended for pregnant females. Women of childbearing age are instructed to prevent pregnancy for three months following rubella injection, as there is a theoretical risk to the unborn child, although no cases of birth defects have been found in women who received rubella immunization just before or during pregnancy. There is no risk to the pregnant woman who is in contact with a child who has received the MMR. Women can have a rubella titer blood test done, which measures the amount of rubella antibodies and tells if they are immune to the disease. This is routinely done in pregnancy, and a rubella vaccine is administered to nonimmune women after delivery.

However, it is best to have the test done prior to becoming pregnant the first time; you may want to consider having it done for your teenage daughter during a regular physical exam.

Haemophilus Influenzae Type B

Haemophilus influenzae type b causes many cases of serious disease in children, most notably meningitis, or inflammation of membranes in the brain and spinal cord. Meningitis is a serious disease and can even lead to death. Haemophilus influenzae can also cause pneumonia and other respiratory diseases, and middle ear infections (otitis media). The diseases caused by Haemophilus influenzae are commonly seen in young children. Some groups acquire more cases of the diseases; these include children from lower socio-economic groups and children with existing diseases such as aplastic anemia, Hodgkin's disease, and sickle cell disease. Healthy children who attend day care or nursery school have been shown to be much more likely to acquire a Haemophilus influenzae disease.

The vaccine for Haemophilus influenzae type b is the newest of the regularly scheduled immunizations, first recommended for all children in 1985. It is injected into subcutaneous tissue, usually in the upper, outer arm and given at two years of age. Children at risk of developing the disease may be immunized at eighteen months. It is not yet known if they will require reimmunization after their second birthday. The vaccine is not effective for children under eighteen months.

Since Haemophilus influenzae type b vaccine is relatively new, your child may not have had it at the age of two years. If your child is under six years of age, contact your health care provider to obtain the vaccine. The vaccine is not routinely given after six years since the incidence of Haemophilus influenzae disease is low in older children. However, if your child is older but may be at risk because of a chronic disease such as immune deficiency, sickle cell disease, Hodgkin's disease, or aplastic anemia, contact your health care provider for advice.

Unintended Effects

Redness or hardness at the injection site and a slight fever for twenty-four hours are sometimes observed after Haemophilus influenzae type b vaccine administration. The side effects are mild and of short duration. The vaccine is not recommended for pregnant women, nursing mothers, or children under eighteen months.

Tuberculosis Testing (TB Test)

Although it is not an immunization, testing for tuberculosis is usually done during well-child health visits. A small amount of derivative from tuberculosis protein is injected just under the skin of the forearm by needle or with a small round cylinder with sharp prongs at the end. If your child has been exposed to tuberculosis, antibodies will be present and a reddened, raised area results from this injection. The area of injection needs to be examined for reaction by you or the health care provider within forty-eight to seventy-two hours after the test. If you are looking for the reaction, be sure to note when the area should be examined and what to look for (usually a hardened, raised area). If there is no reaction, the test is called negative. If there is a reaction, the test is called positive. Anyone who has had a positive test should never receive another TB test; a positive reaction will always occur and can be uncomfortable. Positive reactions are followed by either a different type of TB test or a chest X-ray to be sure there is no active tuberculosis. A positive TB test does not necessarily mean that your child has tuberculosis but rather that exposure to the disease has occurred sometime and antibodies have been produced to fight it.

Tuberculosis testing is usually done at one year of age and every one to two years after that, the schedule depending somewhat on the number of tuberculosis cases in your community. The TB test is not known to have any side effects.

Other Immunizations

As stated previously, smallpox has been totally eradicated worldwide, so immunization for that disease is no longer required. Immunization for other diseases such as yellow fever, cholera, and typhoid may be needed for foreign travel. Influenza vaccines are recommended for some children with chronic diseases but are not routinely given to all children. Rabies vaccine is available for use when someone is exposed to that disease. Some immunizations should not be given to pregnant women because they can harm the unborn child, so inform health care providers prior to immunization if you are pregnant. If your child must receive any immunizations in addition to those that are normally recommended, ask your health care provider for a full explanation of possible unintended effects and their treatment.

PART THREE

*Nonprescription
Medicines*

CHAPTER **6**

Medicines for Fever, Pain, and Inflammation

When people are asked which medicine they take most often or which they administer to their children most often, aspirin or acetaminophen is a likely answer. Both these drugs provide relief from mild pain, whether it be headache, muscular pain, or menstrual cramps, and both reduce the elevated temperatures that accompany colds and other infections. Since pain and fever are frequent symptoms of many minor illnesses, it is no wonder that these medicines are so commonly used for treatment.

Fever

Children's temperatures vary depending on activity, fluid intake, and presence of infection. Children experience fever often because they tend to get many minor illnesses and also because their temperature regulating mechanisms, both in the brain and in the fluid-regulation of the body, are immature. Mild or moderate fever by itself is not a reason for alarm. Assess your child for other symptoms. Is your child listless, cranky, or tired? Is he or she refusing food and drink? Is there any vomiting and/or diarrhea? Is there a cough or wheezing? If fever and other symptoms are mild, the likely cause is a mild viral illness that will be over in one to three days. Moderate or very high fever often accompany bacterial or other illnesses, which require treatment by your health care provider. Although fever is an indication that something is wrong and may need attention, it may require treatment itself since it causes discomfort, disrupts body fluid balance, and can even bring about a convulsion (febrile seizure). Home treatment of fever is discussed here.

Taking a Temperature

If you suspect fever, accurately assess the temperature using one of several methods. Take a temperature when your child has been engaged in quiet activity for about thirty minutes; after vigorous play the temperature may be higher solely due to activity.

Shake a mercury thermometer downward vigorously so the mercury is well below the normal temperature reading, 98.6° F (see Appendix 2 for fahrenheit to centigrade temperature conversions). An easy and accurate way to take the temperature at all ages is the axillary method. Place a thermometer into the underarm very close to the body and securely hold the child's arm against the body for ten minutes. You can rock and sing to the infant or read to the toddler and preschooler during this time. The normal axillary temperature is usually about 97.7° F, or one degree lower than the normal oral temperature.

You may take an oral temperature if your child is old enough to hold the thermometer securely under the tongue without biting down. This is difficult for children younger than five to six years. Wait at least fifteen minutes after your child has had food or drink to take an oral temperature and leave the thermometer under the tongue for three to five minutes. The usual oral temperature is 98.6° F or up to a degree or two higher for the infant and toddler.

When taking a rectal temperature, place your child on the stomach or lift the legs up while the child lies on the back so the rectal opening can be viewed (see page 86). Lubricate the end of the thermometer with a water-soluble lubricant, such as K-Y jelly, and gently insert it about one-half to one inch into the rectum. Hold the thermometer in place for three minutes. It is important to hold the thermometer and prevent the child from turning to avoid breaking the thermometer and harming his or her rectum. The normal rectal temperature is 99.6° F, or one degree more than the normal oral temperature.

There are different types of thermometers for different uses. Rectal thermometers have a round tip to prevent damage to the rectum, while oral thermometers have a longer tip. Either kind may be used for axillary temperatures.

Electronic thermometers are also available; their cost is generally not warranted for home use. Sensor tapes, which can be placed on the forehead or abdomen to give a temperature reading, may be purchased

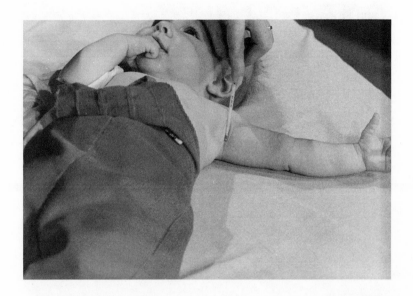

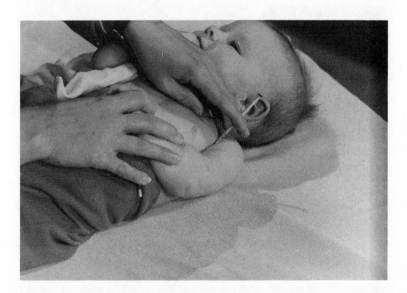

To take a child's temperature by the axillary method, place the thermometer very close to the body against the underarm. Fold the child's arm against his body and hold it there securely for ten minutes. An axillary temperature is usually one degree lower than the oral temperature. *(Roy Ramsey)*

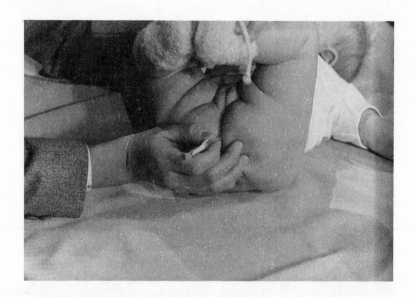

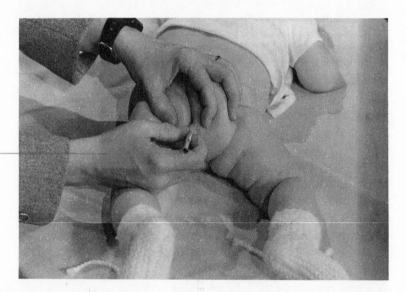

A rectal temperature reading can be taken with the child lying on either her stomach or back with her legs lifted. Once the anus is visible, insert a rectal thermometer, the end of which has been lubricated with a water-soluble lubricant, one-half to one inch into the rectum. Hold it in place for three minutes. A rectal temperature is usually one degree higher than the oral temperature. *(Roy Ramsey)*

in most pharmacies but are not usually as accurate as mercury thermometers.

Clean glass thermometers after use by washing it with lukewarm, not hot, soapy water, drying it, and wiping it with alcohol. Store it in a cool, dry place and wipe it with water or alcohol again prior to its next use. If your mercury thermometer breaks, discard the glass and contents carefully. The amount of mercury contained in a thermometer is not enough to cause concern; however, it does vaporize, so it should be discarded. Consult your Poison Control Center for instructions on the disposal of mercury.

Treatment of Fever

If the temperature is elevated at least two degrees above normal, you can use medicine (aspirin or acetaminophen) and other treatment to reduce fever. (See Table 2 for a list of common aspirin and acetaminophen preparations.) Dress your feverish child in light clothes. Do not use blankets, sweaters, or other heavy clothes. Provide just enough clothing to prevent shivering, since that increases the temperature further. Usually a diaper or underpants and shirt are sufficient for a young child.

Bathing or sponging your child in lukewarm bathwater can also help to lower fever. The water should run over the groin and underarms, where there are large blood supplies. Bathe the child for twenty minutes and repeat again in two hours if needed. However, if shivering begins in the bath, remove and dry the child, and give the bath later after shivering stops. Avoid ice water or alcohol baths, since they cause great discomfort and can be harmful to your child. Alcohol fumes are dangerous for the child to inhale.

Massage may also be helpful in lowering the temperature since it helps dilate blood vessels. Massaging with lotion further enhances the cooling effect, but once again, avoid using alcohol.

Since the feverish child often is nauseated or not hungry, offer your child clear fluids often. These include apple juice, gelatin, ginger ale, popsicles, or other fluids you can see through.

It is important to treat fevers, but it is also often necessary to deal with the underlying cause. If a fever accompanies an ear infection, the child should receive an antibiotic as well as a fever reducer. When the cause is a minor illness such as a mild cold, you can treat the problem at home, but contact your health care provider if the child's fever and illness do not respond to home measures in about two days.

◀ Contact a health care provider if the temperature:

- is above 103° F
- is not lowered by medicine and other measures
- continues for more than two days
- recurs two or more times a few days apart
- is accompanied by other symptoms, such as profuse vomiting, listlessness, irritability, decreased urination, and refusal to drink

Pain

Many of the illnesses that produce fever also create discomfort or mild pain. Fortunately the same nonprescription drugs can be used to treat both these symptoms. Aspirin and acetaminophen decrease the discom-

Table 2 Common Aspirin and Acetaminophen Preparations

Medicine	Active Ingredient	Forms	Dosage
Arthropan	Choline salicylate (an aspirinlike substance)	Liquid	870 mg/5 ml (1 tsp)
Ascriptin	Aspirin buffered with aluminum magnesium hydroxide	Tablet	325 mg (5 gr)
Aspergum	Aspirin	Chewable gum	210 mg
Children's Aspirin*	Aspirin	Tablet	65–81 mg
Bufferin	Aspirin buffered with magnesium carbonate and aluminum glycinate	Tablet	325 mg
Datril	Acetaminophen	Tablet	500 mg
Liquiprin*	Acetaminophen	Liquid	80 mg/1.66 ml (1 dropper)
Panadol	Acetaminophen	Capsule Tablet	500 mg
Phenaphen	Acetaminophen	Capsule	325 mg
Tempra*	Acetaminophen	Syrup	120 mg/5 ml (1 tsp)
		Drops	80 mg/0.8 ml (1 dropper)
Children's Tylenol*	Acetaminophen	Chewable tablet	80 mg
		Elixir	160 mg/5 ml (1 tsp)
		Drops	80 mg/0.8 ml (1 dropper)

* Preparation specifically intended for children.

fort of scraped skin, an immunization, a cold, and many other problems. Once again, it is important to seek medical advice if the pain persists for more than a few days or if the medicines administered at home are not helpful in alleviating the pain. There are prescription medicines such as codeine that can be obtained for severe pain. For a detailed description of codeine, see Chapter 16.

Inflammation

Injuries such as muscle pulls, bruises, or scrapes may cause swelling, redness, and pain at the site. These symptoms are produced by an increased blood flow to the injured area. While some increase in blood flow is helpful to ensure fast healing, excess causes pain and actually impedes the flow of nutrients to and waste products from cells, thereby slowing the healing process. Aspirin, one of the medicines used to treat fever and pain, decreases inflammation as well, while acetaminophen does not. Aspirin is thus the medicine of choice when pain is accompanied by inflammation. An additional medicine, ibuprofen, was more recently approved for the nonprescription treatment of pain. This medicine is particularly effective in treating inflammatory problems.

ACETAMINOPHEN

Trade Names: Aspirin Free Anacin, Bromo-Seltzer, Co-Tylenol, Datril, Excedrin, Liquiprin, Panadol, Phenaphen, Tempra, Tylenol.

Dosage Forms: Tablets (regular and chewable), drops, elixir.

Why Used: Acetaminophen is used as an analgesic to reduce mild to moderate pain and as an antipyretic to reduce fever. Its potency and action are similar to that of aspirin.

How to Give: Place drops in the mouth or have the child drink the elixir from the accompanying cup. Chewable tablets are chewed and followed with water. Give regular tablets with a generous amount of water.

Unintended Effects: Acetaminophen is generally believed to have no side effects when taken in recommended dosages.

Drug and Food Interactions: None known.

Contraindications: Acetaminophen is contraindicated in a child with liver disease and the rare child who shows hypersensitivity to this medicine.

Special Notes:

- There are two forms of liquid acetaminophen. One is an elixir and contains 120 mg of medicine in 5 ml of liquid, while the other is in the form of drops and contains 80 mg in 0.8 ml of liquid. Read labels carefully to avoid administering an incorrect dosage of medicine.
- The drug is broken down by the liver, so it can accumulate to toxic levels if given to a child with liver disease.
- Acetaminophen is combined with other drugs such as aspirin by some manufacturers. These products are usually more expensive and have not been shown to be more effective than single ingredient preparation.
- The drug is harmful if taken in excess. Keep it locked out of reach of children and contact the Poison Control Center immediately if your child gets an excessive dose.

Age Limitations: Some packages do not have dosages for children under two years. Contact your health care provider for correct dosage if this happens.

Storage Instructions: Keep at room temperature.

ASPIRIN (ACETYLSALICYLIC ACID)

Trade Names: Alka-Seltzer, Anacin, A.S.A., Ascriptin, Aspergum, Bufferin, Ecotrin, Encaprin, Empirin.

Dosage Forms: Tablet (regular, effervescent, enteric coated, chewable, and time release), rectal suppository, chewing gum.

Why Used: Aspirin is a salicylate product that is effective as an analgesic to reduce mild to moderate pain, as an antipyretic to reduce fever, and as an antiinflammatory to reduce swelling and discomfort.

How to Give: Give tablets with a generous amount of water. Be sure rectum is free of stool if administering rectal suppository.

Unintended Effects:

- Aspirin commonly causes stomach distress, burning, nausea, and vomiting; more rarely, bleeding and ulcers.
- Aspirin alters the platelets of the blood, increasing chances of bleeding throughout the body. The newborn baby's ability to clot blood is affected if the mother takes aspirin in late pregnancy.
- Occasionally children are allergic to aspirin, showing rash or breathing difficulty.
- When repeated doses are taken for long periods of time, aspirin can build

up in the body. Symptoms of overdose in such cases are labored breathing, ringing in the ears, headache, stomach distress, bleeding, and agitation. Overdosage with aspirin remains a major source of poisoning for children. This medicine is powerful when taken in excess, causing serious illness and even death. Therefore, purchase aspirin in child-resistant containers and keep it locked out of your child's reach.

- An increase in numbers of cases of Reye's syndrome, a neurological disease, has been noted when young children are treated with aspirin for chickenpox or influenza. In the child with one of these problems, acetaminophen should be given rather than aspirin.

Drug and Food Interactions: Effervescent aspirin (i.e., Alka-Seltzer) is high in sodium, an important factor to consider if the child is on a low-sodium diet.

Aspirin interacts adversely with a number of prescription drugs that are infrequently administered in childhood. However, if your child is taking any prescription medicine(s) or large doses of vitamin C, check with your health care provider before administering aspirin.

Contraindications: Aspirin is contraindicated in persons hypersensitive to the medicine, in young children being treated for chickenpox or influenza, in late pregnancy, in those undergoing oral procedures (e.g., tonsillectomy or dental work), and in persons with bleeding disorders or kidney disease. Since it is excreted in breast milk, the nursing mother should minimize its use, although an occasional dose should not harm the nursing baby.

Special Notes:

- Buffered aspirin is a special preparation that helps decrease the stomach irritation common with this medicine. The same effect can be created by administering aspirin with a glass of milk or other snack and is considerably less expensive than purchasing buffered or enteric-coated aspirin.
- Generic aspirin has not been shown to be less effective than trade brands and thus can be safely and effectively used.
- Time-release preparations have not been demonstrated to provide longer duration of action; neither do they minimize unintended effects. Their absorption rate is quite variable.
- Aspirin is available in combination preparations with other products such as caffeine. The effectiveness of these products has not been demonstrated and the resulting combinations are often much more expensive than aspirin alone. Read labels carefully.
- Aspirin dosage is often labeled in grains (gr), and since 1 grain is the same as 60 to 65 milligrams (mg), the adult aspirin tablets commonly

used each contain 5 gr or 325 mg. Children's aspirin is available in 1 gr (60 mg) and 1¼ gr (80 mg) tablets.

- Rectal suppositories can irritate the lining of the rectum and their absorption may be unpredictable, so tablets are recommended unless your child is vomiting. Tablets can be crushed and administered with a small amount of food for easy swallowing. Children's chewable tablets are also available.
- The chewing gum with aspirin (Aspergum) is often irritating to the inside of the mouth. If this should occur, discontinue use. Aspirin tablets will be just as effective, even to treat discomfort in the throat.

Age Limitations: Consult your health care provider before administering the rectal suppository to children under four years. Consult your health care provider for proper dosage in children under two years.

Storage Instructions: Keep at room temperature with cover tightly closed.

IBUPROFEN

Trade Names: Advil, Nuprin.

Dosage Form: Tablet.

Why Used: Ibuprofen is used as an analgesic to reduce mild to moderate pain and to decrease the swelling of inflammation. It also helps to reduce fever. Potency and action are similar to aspirin.

How to Give: Give with a generous amount of water.

Unintended Effects: Upset stomach or heartburn may occur.

Drug and Food Interactions: Use with caution if anticoagulants are also being administered.

Contraindications: Do not give this drug to children under twelve years without the advice of a health care provider. Do not give if your child has been hypersensitive to other nonprescription pain relievers. It is contraindicated in late pregnancy.

Special Notes:

- This drug has been available with prescription and was approved for nonprescription use in 1984. It has not been widely tested in young children yet; thus the caution not to administer to children under twelve years.

- If the painful area becomes increasingly swollen or red, see a health care provider.
- This drug should not be taken at the same time as aspirin or acetaminophen unless directed to do so by your health care provider.
- Keep this drug locked out of reach of your children.

Age Limitations: Do not give to children under twelve years without the advice of a health care provider.

Storage Instructions: Keep at room temperature.

CHAPTER 7

Vitamins and Minerals

Vitamins are chemical substances that are essential in small amounts for the efficient and optimal utilization of ingested food by the body. The body cannot produce or synthesize vitamins. They have to come from external sources—our daily diet. Vitamins need a suitable environment in which to operate; they are of no value to the body in the absence of protein, fat, carbohydrates, water, and oxygen.

Many health professionals believe that for a normal child, additional intake of vitamins besides those present in a well-balanced diet is an unnecessary expense. However, there are exceptions. Dieting and reduced food consumption have become a national obsession, especially among teenagers. Vitamins and minerals have specific indications for those who are on a restricted diet. Athletes, especially adolescent athletes who are in training for competitive physical activities; babies whose diet consists predominantly of dairy products or infant formulas; and children who are growing rapidly all may need the supplemental action of vitamins. If you have any questions about whether your child should take supplemental vitamins or minerals, you can use the Recommended Daily Allowances (RDAs) as a guideline (see Table 3) and discuss your concerns with your health care provider.

The RDAs are established by the National Research Council and the Food and Nutrition Board of the National Academy of Sciences. They are designed for the maintenance of good nutrition of healthy individuals of different age groups in the United States, with provisions for variations among most normal persons under usual environmental stress. The values specified are not requirements; they are recommended

Table 3 Recommended Daily Allowances (RDAs) of Vitamins and Minerals

Age (years)	Thiamine (B_1, mg)	Riboflavin (B_2, mg)	Niacin (B_3, mg)	Pyridoxine (B_6, mg)	Cyanocobalamine (B_{12}, mcg)	Folic Acid (mcg)	Ascorbic Acid (mg)	A (IU)	D (IU)	E (IU)	K (mcg)	Calcium (mg)	Iron (mg)	Zinc (mg)
Birth–0.5	0.3	0.4	6	0.3	0.5	30	35	1400	400	4.5	12	360	10	3
0.5–1	0.5	0.6	8	0.6	1.5	45	35	2000	400	6	10–20	540	15	5
1–3	0.7	0.8	9	0.9	2	100	45	2000	400	7.5	15–30	800	15	10
4–6	0.9	1.0	11	1.3	2.5	200	45	2500	400	9	20–40	800	15	10
7–10	1.2	1.4	16	1.6	3	300	45	3300	400	10.5	30–60	800	10	10
Males { 11–14	1.4	1.7	18	1.8	3	400	50	5000	400	12	50–100	1200	18	15
15–18	1.4	1.8	18	2.0	3	400	60	5000	400	15	50–100	1200	18	15
Females { 11–14	1.1	1.3	15	1.8	3	400	50	4000	400	12	50–100	1200	18	15
15–18	1.1	1.3	14	2.0	3	400	60	4000	400	12	50–100	1200	18	15

Reproduced from *Recommended Dietary Allowances*, 9th Edition (1980), with the permission of the National Academy of Sciences, Washington, D.C.

daily intakes of certain essential nutrients. Based on current knowledge, they are believed to be adequate for the energy needs of healthy individuals and are not intended to cover therapeutic nutritional requirements in disease or other abnormal states.

Several terms that frequently appear on vitamin bottles or advertisements need some explanation here. These are: *organic, natural,* and *synthetic.* Organic denotes originating from living substances such as plants, animals, or microorganisms. Natural implies deriving from nature's sources rather than artificial fabrication. Most vitamins are extracted from natural sources, such as cod liver and rose hips, the fleshy fruit of a rose, but such natural sources are relatively limited, and it is impractical to rely solely on them for the abundant supply of these drugs (yes, vitamins are drugs) that line the shelves of health food stores, pharmacies, and discount and variety stores. Hence, it is inevitable that vitamins have to be synthesized or manufactured chemically. Such a method of manufacturing does not make synthetic vitamins any less inferior in quality to the natural or organic vitamins since pharmaceutical companies are required to comply with guidelines established by the U.S. Food and Drug Administration. Synthetic vitamins are effective and can usually be produced at costs lower than natural ones. Therefore, it is difficult to justify the high price of vitamins branded organic or natural.

Many vitamins are surprisingly safe, as the following discussion shows. They may, however, foster a false sense of psychological relief. Rather than seeking remedies in vitamins because your child has experienced fatigue, weakness, pale color, lack of energy, loss of appetite or weight, you are better off consulting a health professional regarding these symptoms.

During the past decade huge doses of vitamins, called megavitamins, have been advocated for the treatment of mental illness, learning disabilities, and even malignancy. There is no scientific evidence to support these claims. The American Academy of Pediatrics does not recommend vitamin supplements beyond the vitamins to be found in a well-balanced diet. The American Pediatric Association has also condemned megavitamin therapy. If you believe that megavitamin therapy would be beneficial for your child, discuss the pros and cons with your health care provider and read the current theories on this subject before making a decision. If you use megavitamins, carefully observe your child for symptoms of excessive intake, which are many and varied, depending on the vitamin which is in excess. These symptoms are described in this chapter under the respective vitamins and minerals.

Since vitamins are present in all foods and needed for all ages, information on Drug and Food Interactions and Age Limitation is not applicable here. The Recommended Daily Allowances as well as manufacturer's recommendations on the drug label should, therefore, serve as guidelines and instructions for use unless otherwise specified by your health care provider.

Vitamins

VITAMIN A

Trade Names: Alphalin, Aquasol A, Sust-A, Vitamin A.

Major Dietary Sources: Eggs, liver, meats, yellow vegetables, fruits, butterfat and milk products.

Dosage Forms: Tablet, capsule, drop, injection.

Function: Essential for the retina of the eye (for night vision), growth, cell and bone development.

Symptoms of Deficiency: Dry eyes, dry skin, night-blindness, sensitivity of the eye to light, faulty bone formation, reduced resistance to infection, and retarded growth.

RDAs:		
	birth to 6 months	1400 IU
	6 months to 1 year	2000 IU
	1 to 3 years	2000 IU
	4 to 6 years	2500 IU
	7 to 10 years	3300 IU

Unintended Effects: Intake in excess of body requirement results in a condition known as hypervitaminosis A. Symptoms are fatigue; loss of appetite; irritability; headache; bulging forehead, especially in a young child; joint and muscle pain; swollen and tender arms and legs; dry and cracked skin; abdominal discomfort.

Drug and Food Interactions: Mineral oil reduces the absorption of vitamin A in the intestine.

Contraindication: Existing condition of hypervitaminosis A.

Special Notes:

- By convention, dosages of vitamin A are measured in International Units (IU) rather than milligrams.
- Any excessive intake of this vitamin is stored in the liver. The normal adult liver storage is sufficient to satisfy two years' requirements of vitamin A. Therefore, unintended effects become evident when the accumulation in the body exceeds the saturation level.
- If, judging from your dietary practice, you decide that your child is not getting sufficient vitamin A, consult your health care provider. Overzealous feeding with fish liver oil or chicken liver can induce hypervitaminosis A. Self-medication with vitamin A or multivitamin products that contain a large dose of vitamin A (above 5000 IU) is potentially harmful.
- Fat malabsorption or insufficient secretion of bile or pancreatic enzyme results in vitamin A deficiency.
- Topical application of vitamin A (retinoic acid) is sometimes prescribed for acne. It works for some but not for others. The formulation of retinoic acid is different from oral vitamin A. It is a different drug altogether, so vitamin A oral liquid cannot be used on acne. Other claims, such as wound healing and treatment of burns, are not substantiated by research evidence.

Storage Instruction: Keep at room temperature unless the gelatinlike capsules stick together, then keep them in a cool dry place.

VITAMIN B₁ (THIAMINE)

Trade Names: Betalin S, Bewon, Pan-B-1, Thiamine.

Major Dietary Sources: Unrefined cereal and rice grains, pork, beef, fresh peas.

Dosage Forms: Tablet, elixir, injection.

Function: Essential for carbohydrate metabolism.

Symptoms of Deficiency: Deficiency affects the heart and nervous system and is manifest in swelling and numbness of the extremities, increased heart rate, and muscle weakness.

RDAs:		
	birth to 6 months	0.3 mg
	6 months to 1 year	0.5 mg
	1 to 3 years	0.7 mg
	4 to 6 years	0.9 mg
	7 to 10 years	1.2 mg

Unintended Effects: None from the oral intake of this vitamin. Thiamine is not accumulated in the body.

Contraindication: None.

Special Notes:

- Thiamine deficiency is rare. Increase in metabolic rate or prolonged stomach disturbances such as diarrhea or malabsorption may necessitate increased thiamine intake. Poor dietary habits, alcoholism, and pregnancy also increase the likelihood of thiamine deficiency.
- When intake exceeds the minimal requirement, the body's tissue stores become saturated. Any excess quantity is excreted in the urine.

Storage Instruction: Keep at room temperature.

VITAMIN B₂ (RIBOFLAVIN)

Trade Name: Riboflavin.

Major Dietary Sources: Eggs, meat, milk, fish, liver, whole grain cereals, and green vegetables.

Dosage Forms: Tablet, injection.

Function: Essential for cell growth and tissue replacement.

Symptoms of Deficiency: Sores on the tongue, the lips, and the face; itching and burning of the eye; sensitivity of the eye to light; flaky skin, especially in skin folds; and diminished visual acuity.

RDAs:		
	birth to 6 months	0.4 mg
	6 months to 1 year	0.6 mg
	1 to 3 years	0.8 mg
	4 to 6 years	1.0 mg
	7 to 10 years	1.4 mg

Unintended Effects: None. Riboflavin is not accumulated in the body.

Contraindication: None.

Special Note: Any intake above the minimal requirement is excreted in the urine.

Storage Instruction: Keep at room temperature.

VITAMIN B₃ (NICOTINIC ACID OR NIACIN)

Trade Names: Nicotinex, Nicotinic Acid (Niacin), SK-Niacin, Span-Niacin-150.

Major Dietary Sources: Yeast, lean meat, liver, eggs, and peanuts.

Dosage Forms: Tablet, elixir, injection.

Function: Essential for protein metabolism.

Symptoms of Deficiency: Skin eruptions, excessive saliva, red and swollen tongue which may break out in sores, water or bloody diarrhea, nausea and vomiting, headache, dizziness, insomnia, and hallucinations.

RDAs:		
	birth to 6 months	6 mg
	6 months to 1 year	8 mg
	1 to 3 years	9 mg
	4 to 6 years	11 mg
	7 to 10 years	16 mg

Unintended Effects:

- May upset stomach.
- Produces a sensation of warmth; a flush especially around the neck, ears, and face; headache; and tingling of the lips.
- Occasionally results in skin rash, itching.

Contraindication: Existing liver disease.

Special Notes:

- Any excessive intake above the body's requirement is excreted in the urine.
- The unintended effects usually disappear with continued intake.
- There is no evidence that large doses of niacin are effective in treating psychotic disorder, as has been claimed by some medical practitioners.
- Doses above 100 mg and sustained-release capsules require prescription.
- Nicotinamide is a different chemical form from nicotinic acid or niacin, but the body uses it as a source of the vitamin. The advantage of nicotinamide over the other two is that it does not produce the flushing sensation.

Storage Instruction: Keep at room temperature.

VITAMIN B₆ (PYRIDOXINE)

Trade Names: Hexa-Betalin, Pan-B-6, Pyridoxine, TexSix T.R.

Major Dietary Sources: Meat, whole grain cereals, lentils, nuts, bananas, avocados, potatoes and green vegetables.

Dosage Forms: Tablet, sustained-release capsule, injection.

Function: Essential for the metabolism of protein, fat, and carbohydrate.

Symptoms of Deficiency: Flaky skin patches about the eyes, nose, and mouth accompanied by sores of the tongue and inside the mouth, and numbness of the extremities. Extreme deficiency in infants can result in seizures.

RDAs:		
	birth to 6 months	0.3 mg
	6 months to 1 year	0.6 mg
	1 to 3 years	0.9 mg
	4 to 6 years	1.3 mg
	7 to 10 years	1.6 mg

Unintended Effects: Rare.

Contraindication: None.

Special Notes:

- Infants generally obtain vitamin B₆ from breast milk or formula. However, if the breast-feeding mother has a low level of vitamin B₆ herself or if the infant does not have adequate intake from formula, deficiency results, although this is rare.
- Injection is usually given when severe deficiency is diagnosed, especially if the child develops seizures.

Storage Instruction: Keep tablets at room temperature.

VITAMIN B₁₂ (CYANOCOBALAMINE)

Trade Names: Kaybovite, Redisol, Vitamin B₁₂.

Major Dietary Sources: Liver, kidney, shellfish, meat, fish, eggs, and milk.

Dosage Forms: Regular and soluble tablet, capsule, injection.

Function: Essential for fat and carbohydrate metabolism, especially in cell reproduction and growth.

Symptoms of Deficiency: Sore mouth, tingling and numbness of the extremities progressing to poor muscular coordination, unsteadiness, mental slowness, agitation, hallucinations, anemia, and dim vision.

RDAs:	birth to 6 months	0.5 mcg
	6 months to 1 year	1.5 mcg
	1 to 3 years	2.0 mcg
	4 to 6 years	2.5 mcg
	7 to 10 years	3.0 mcg

Unintended Effects: None.

Contraindication: None.

Special Notes:

- The dietary absorption of cyanocobalamine in a child with short bowel syndrome, prolonged diarrhea, or other absorption abnormalities may not be reliable nor adequate. Hence vitamin B_{12} supplement, preferably in injection form, is recommended.
- Infants generally obtain vitamin B_{12} from breast milk or formula. If the breast-feeding mother has a low level of vitamin B_{12}, such as in the case of someone adhering to a strict vegetarian diet, her child should receive supplement by injection.
- Taking folic acid supplement may correct the anemia induced by vitamin B_{12} deficiency but not the neurological symptoms associated with it. The indiscriminate use of folic acid, therefore, can mask the anemia and delay the diagnosis of vitamin B_{12} deficiency since anemia is more easily identified than the neurological symptoms.
- The body recycles vitamin B_{12} efficiently, so in some cases deficiency may take a few years to manifest symptomatically. Therefore, it is advisable to investigate the reasons for malabsorption of vitamin B_{12}; any "shotgun" approach—a vitamin B_{12} injection—may delay the discovery of some underlying disorder.

Storage Instruction: The injection is kept refrigerated if to be administered at home. Keep the tablet at room temperature.

VITAMIN C (ASCORBIC ACID)

Trade Names: Ascorbic Acid, Cevalin, Cevita, Flavorcee, Vitacee, Viterra C.

Major Dietary Sources: Fruits (especially citrus, e.g., oranges, grapefruits) and vegetables (e.g., tomatoes).

Dosage Forms: Regular, chewable and sustained-release tablet, sustained-release capsule, drop, injection.

Function: Essential for carbohydrate metabolism and the makeup of bone and connective tissues.

Symptoms of Deficiency: Degenerative changes in blood vessels, bone, and connective tissues (scurvy); impaired wound healing; joint and muscle aches; weakness; loss of appetite; bleeding abnormalities; and swollen gums.

RDAs:

	birth to 1 year	35 mg
	1 to 10 years	45 mg

Unintended Effects: High doses of vitamin C taken by mouth may lead to the development of stones in the urinary tract as well as diarrhea.

Drug and Food Interactions: Ascorbic acid increases the absorption of iron and aspirin but accelerates the excretion of the prescription medicine imipramine. Consult the pharmacist for other possible interactions between vitamin C and other medicines used for chronic illnesses, such as imipramine for enuresis, aspirin for arthritis, and dextroamphetamine for Attention Deficit Disorder.

Contraindication: Previous allergy to vitamin C.

Special Notes:

- Vitamin C is destroyed by heating and excessive cooking. Although the ready-to-use, commercial infant formulas may already be fortified with vitamin C, the amount present may partially be destroyed by heating during manufacturing. Consult your health care provider for the need of vitamin C supplement if your child is strictly on a formula diet.
- Some researchers have claimed that vitamin C decreases the incidence and duration of the common cold and other illnesses. However, these claims have not been substantiated by many studies.
- Large doses of vitamin C may give a false negative reading in urine testing with Tes-Tape and Clinistix and a false positive reading with Clinitest.

Storage Instruction: Keep at room temperature.

VITAMIN D (ERGOCALCIFEROL)

Trade Names: Calciferol, Deltalin, Drisdol, Vitamin D.

Major Dietary Sources: Fish liver oil, milk products, and cereals.

Dosage Forms: Capsule, tablet, liquid, injection.

Function: Essential for calcium absorption, which is needed for bone development.

Symptoms of Deficiency: Rickets or defective bone growth.

RDAs: birth to 10 years   400 IU

Unintended Effects: Excessive intake of vitamin D leads to an elevated level of calcium in the body, which results in loss of appetite, nausea, fatigue, weakness, weight loss, aches and stiffness, constipation and diarrhea. If the condition continues, damage to the blood vessels, brain, kidney, and heart occurs as a result of calcium deposits.

Drug and Food Interactions:

- Mineral oil reduces absorption of vitamin D.
- A child who takes phenytoin or phenobarbital for treatment of seizures may need vitamin D supplement, because these two drugs affect vitamin D metabolism in the body and may produce a low calcium level. Consult your health care provider on the need for vitamin D supplement.

Contraindications:

- Existing elevated level of calcium in the body (hypercalcemia).
- Existing elevated level of phosphate in the body (hyperphosphatemia).

Special Notes:

- With the advent of the addition of vitamin D to food products such as milk, bread, and cereals, the individual child's intake of this vitamin varies. Since the body utilizes sunlight to make vitamin D, the extent of exposure to sunlight poses another variable in the body's levels of vitamin D. In general, vitamin D supplement is recommended for infants and children; however, it should be given after scrutiny of the diet and with guidance from the health care provider.
- Liver disease impairs the absorption of vitamin D from the digestive tract. Kidney disease would affect calcium metabolism, which is made possible by vitamin D. Thus various preparations of vitamin D are available for children with specific needs.
- Vitamin D as a single drug requires prescription, but it is a common ingredient in multivitamin products. Be sure to read the label to make sure your child is not taking an excessive dose.
- The dosage of vitamin D is measured in International Units (IU) rather than milligrams.

Storage Instruction: Keep at room temperature unless the gelatinlike capsules stick together, then keep them in a cool dry place.

VITAMIN E

Trade Names: Aquasol E, Cen-E, D-Alpha-E, Dalfatol, E-Ferol, Eprolin, Epsilan-M, Solucap E, Tocopher-M, Vitamin E, Vita-Plus E.

Major Dietary Sources: Vegetable oils (e.g., wheat germ oil, margarine, shortening), leafy vegetables, whole grains, cereals, milk, eggs, and meats.

Dosage Forms: Capsule, chewable and regular tablet, drop.

Function: Preserves integrity of cell walls and protects them from breakdown by oxygen.

Symptoms of Deficiency: Anemia and swelling of extremities.

RDAs:		
	birth to 6 months	4.5 IU
	6 months to 1 year	6.0 IU
	1 to 3 years	7.5 IU
	4 to 6 years	9.0 IU
	7 to 10 years	10.5 IU

Unintended Effects: None.

Contraindication: None.

Special Notes:

- Requirement of vitamin E increases with the intake of polyunsaturated fats, especially in low birth weight premature infants.
- If you have any reason to suspect that your infant or child has inadequate intake of vitamin E in the diet, consult your health care provider about the need for a vitamin E supplement.
- Swelling in an infant can be a symptom of a variety of disorders. It is inadvisable to begin treatment of swelling with vitamin E on your own without consulting your health care provider.
- Fat malabsorption impedes the body's absorption of vitamin E.
- Despite the relative safety of this drug, supplemental intake can be an unnecessary expense.

Storage Instruction: Keep at room temperature unless the gelatinlike capsules stick together, then keep them in a cool dry place.

VITAMIN K

Trade Names: Aqua-Mephyton, Kappadione, Mephyton, Synkavite.

Major Dietary Sources: Green vegetables, dairy products, fruits, and cereals.

Dosage Forms: Tablet, injection.

Function: Essential for the formation of blood-clotting factors.

Symptoms of Deficiency: Bleeding.

RDAs:		
	Birth to 6 months	12 mcg
	6 months to 1 year	10–20 mcg
	1 to 3 years	15–30 mcg
	4 to 6 years	20–40 mcg
	7 to 10 years	30–60 mcg

Unintended Effects:

- Allergic reactions, such as skin rash and hives.
- May occasionally upset stomach.

Contraindication: Use with caution in newborns who have a very high level of bilirubin.

Drug and Food Interactions: Mineral oil reduces absorption of vitamin K.

Special Notes:

- Vitamin K is a prescription drug that is not present in multivitamin combination products.
- It is customary to give newborns an injection of vitamin K to prevent bleeding because of the low levels of blood-clotting factors in newborns.
- Malabsorption of the digestive system and liver disorder impede the absorption of vitamin K.
- If an increase in bleeding tendency is suspected, consult your health care provider; it can have numerous causes.

Storage Instruction: Keep tablets at room temperature.

Minerals

CALCIUM

Trade Names: Ca-Plus, Elecal, Florical, Glycate, Neo-Calglucon, Oscal 500.

Major Dietary Sources: Milk and dairy products.

Dosage Forms: Capsule, tablet, powder, syrup, injection.

Function: Necessary for bone growth and teeth. Also essential for blood clotting, integrity of the nervous and muscular systems, and normal heart function.

Symptoms of Deficiency: Deficiency affects the bony structure and functions of the nervous and muscular systems. Symptoms are manifest in bone deformities, inability of the muscle to contract (twitching, tingling spasms), or, in severe cases, seizures.

RDAs:

birth to 6 months	360 mg
6 months to 1 year	540 mg
1 to 10 years	800 mg

Unintended Effects: Constipation; other effects are rare. However, excessive intake of vitamin D can result in elevated levels of calcium in the body (hypercalcemia), which are manifest in constipation, loss of appetite, dry mouth, nausea, vomiting, thirst, and abdominal pain.

Drug and Food Interactions:

- Certain food substances reduce the absorption of calcium; these include rhubarb, spinach, bran, and whole cereals as well as phosphorus, which is present in milk and other dairy products.
- Vitamin D enhances the absorption of calcium; the presence of an excessive amount of vitamin D in the body can also result in hypercalcemia, potentially leading to problems associated with excess calcium, such as deposits in the kidneys, heart, and blood vessels.
- Calcium decreases the absorption of tetracycline; avoid taking both drugs within an hour of each other.

Contraindications: Existing conditions of hypervitaminosis D (excess vitamin D in the body) or hypercalcemia.

Special Notes:

- Due to the large quantity of milk ingested by children in this country, calcium deficiency is rare unless there is abnormal calcium metabolism or milk intolerance; then calcium supplement is indicated.
- Several of the nonprescription digestive aids such as Tums and Camalox contain a significant amount of calcium.
- Calcium comes in different chemical forms: calcium gluconate, calcium lactate, and calcium carbonate. Consult your pharmacist when selecting a supplement for your child.

Storage Instruction: Keep tablets at room temperature.

FLUORIDE

Trade Names: Fluorigard, which does not require a prescription; some prescription products include Flura, Flura-Drops, Flura-Loz, Fluritab, Fluorinse, Cluoral, Pediaflor, Thera-Flur.

Major Dietary Source: Drinking water if it is fluoridated.

Dosage Forms: Liquid, regular and chewable tablet, mouth rinse, gel.

Function: Essential for the formation of strong enamel to prevent dental caries.

Symptoms of Deficiency: Increased incidence of dental caries.

RDAs: Vary with the amount of fluoride already present in drinking water.

Fluoride content of drinking water less than 0.3 ppm

birth to 2 years	0.25 mg
2 to 3 years	0.50 mg
3 to 14 years	1 mg

Fluoride content of drinking water 0.3–0.7 ppm

birth to 2 years	0
2 to 3 years	0.25 mg
3 to 14 years	0.5 mg

Unintended Effects:

- Rarely, allergic reactions such as skin rash, hives, and inflammation.
- Occasionally causes upset stomach.
- Harmful effects from fluoride can occur in one of two ways:

  1. prolonged use of large amount (over 2 mg of fluoride per 2 pints or 1000 cc of drinking water a day during the period of tooth development)
  2. acute ingestion of a large dose (over 200 mg in one dose)

In the former case dental fluorosis results (opaque, white patches scattered unevenly over tooth surfaces). These white patches may become yellowish brown to black-stained pits in more advanced cases. Ingestion of fluoride in amounts of more than 4 to 8 mg per 2 pints or 1000 cc of drinking water can lead to bone cell deformation.

Acute toxicity is manifested by nausea, vomiting, abdominal cramps, diarrhea, shock, and seizure.

Drug and Food Interactions: Dairy products that contain calcium reduce the absorption of fluoride.

Contraindications:

- Previous allergy to fluoride.
- Drinking water with fluoride in excess of 0.7 ppm.

Special Notes:

- There is sufficient clinical evidence to demonstrate the efficacy of adding fluoride to drinking water in the reduction of dental caries. The amount present in most communal drinking water is about 1 mg per 1000 cc (or 2 pints). Taking into consideration an average intake of water, if the water supply is not fluoridated, each child should receive fluoride supplement up to age twelve. Consult the local public health authority or a dentist for the latest recommendation (see Table 4).
- The entire tube of fluoride toothpaste does not contain a dangerous amount of fluoride.
- Fluoride is a prescription drug except when contained in toothpastes and certain brands of mouth rinses.
- Do not eat, drink, or rinse the mouth for fifteen to thirty minutes after fluoride rinses or the application of fluoride gel. Be sure to consult your health care provider on the methods of administering the particular form of fluoride supplement prescribed for your child.

Storage Instruction: Keep at room temperature.

Age Limitations:

- Do not use 1 mg tablets or rinse as a supplement for children under three years or when the fluoride content of drinking water is 0.3 ppm or more,

Table 4   Recommended Fluoride Dose

Fluoride in Water Supply (in parts per million)	Age (years)	Fluoride Dosage (mg/day)
under 0.3 ppm*	Birth–2	0.25
	2–3	0.50
	3–14	1.00
0.3–0.7 ppm	Birth–2	0
	2–3	0.25
	3–14	0.50
over 0.7 ppm	Birth–2	0
	2–3	0
	3–14	0

* 0.3 ppm = 0.3 mg per 1000 cc

unless your health care provider directs otherwise.
- Do not use 1 mg rinses in children under six years unless your health care provider directs otherwise.

IRON

Trade Names: Feosol, Fer-In-Sol, Fergon, Ferrous Sulfate, Ferrous Gluconate, Ferrous Fumarate.

Major Dietary Sources: Present in all types of food. There is an average of 6 mg of iron present in 1000 kcal of the regular American diet. About 20 percent comes from vegetables, 30 to 35 percent from meat, 20 to 25 percent from cereal products. Liver, raisins, and other dried fruits are particularly rich in iron.

Dosage Forms: Liquid, elixir, syrup, regular and sustained-release capsule, regular and sustained-release tablet, injection.

Function: A component of red blood cells, essential for carrying oxygen in blood.

Symptoms of Deficiency: Anemia, which is manifest in fatigue, weakness, lack of energy, impaired learning ability, pale color, increased heart rate, and shortness of breath upon exertion.

RDAs:		
	birth to 6 months	10 mg
	6 months to 1 year	15 mg
	1 to 3 years	15 mg
	4 to 10 years	10 mg

Unintended Effects:
- Commonly causes upset stomach, constipation (or less commonly diarrhea), and black stools.
- May also cause temporary staining of the teeth when the liquid form is taken by mouth.
- Ingestion of large amounts of vitamin tablets containing iron by children happens commonly. Initial symptoms are nausea, vomiting, and bloody diarrhea, followed by lethargy, shock, and depressed respiration. A period of recovery may ensue, only to progress to more life-threatening symptoms later (twelve to forty-eight hours after ingestion) by lack of energy, drop in blood pressure and heart rate, convulsion, and coma.

Drug and Food Interactions:

- Vitamin C enhances iron absorption in the intestine, but antacids reduce iron absorption.
- Iron reduces the absorption of tetracycline; the two drugs should not be taken within two hours of each other.
- Certain food substances, such as milk, eggs, bread, and cereal, also reduce iron absorption.

Contraindications:

- Bleeding disorder of the intestine.
- Previous allergy to tartrazine, which is a dye present in some of the iron tablet coatings or iron liquid.
- Existing blood disorder, a history of or receiving multiple blood transfusions.

Special Notes:

- Iron deficiency is the only specific nutritional deficiency recognized as being prevalent in industrialized nations. Reasons are reduced food intake, obsolescence of iron cooking utensils, increased stature in children (as a result of rapid growth), and early onset of menarche (as a source of blood loss).
- The rapid growth of infants and low iron content of infants' milk diet (approximately 1 mg per 1000 cc or 2 pints) account for widespread iron deficiency in the first two years of life. Appropriate introduction of a varied diet, including iron-fortified cereals, and the routine use of iron supplement either in the form of iron drops or iron-supplemented formula can eliminate this problem. It is advisable to work with your health care provider on a diet plan and nutritional supplement for your child rather than simply purchasing a bottle of iron drops or tablets from a pharmacy and start self-medicating. The mother's iron level during pregnancy will influence the amount of iron stores in the body of the child up to six months of age.
- The predominant reasons for iron deficiency are blood loss and inadequate dietary intake. For the teenage girl, however, menstrual loss is by far the largest determining factor. Thus if your daughter appears to have heavy menstrual loss every month, a blood test can determine the level of red blood cells.
- In the presence of iron deficiency anemia, the body has increased capability to absorb dietary iron.
- The most economic way to take iron supplement, if it is indicated, is to purchase iron tablets alone rather than in combination with other vitamins, which may not be needed. The sustained-release form of iron

tablets or capsules may not be completely absorbed, because they may be transported beyond the section of the gut where maximal iron absorption takes place. Besides, these dosage forms are usually more expensive than the regular tablets or capsules.

- When the liquid form is used, be sure to rinse your child's mouth following ingestion with a full glass of liquid to prevent staining of the teeth.

Storage Instructions: Keep iron tablets and capsules as well as multivitamins containing iron out of your child's reach. An overdose of iron is an emergency. Contact your local Poison Control Center immediately for advice if you suspect your child to have taken iron or iron-containing tablets.

ZINC

Trade Names: Orazinc, Zinc Gluconate, Zinc Sulfate, Zincate, Zinkaps-110, ZNG, Zn-Plus.

Major Dietary Sources: A common substance in every type of food unless an individual is on a chemical diet (feeding by vein).

Dosage Forms: Tablet, capsule.

Function: Essential for protein and carbohydrate metabolism.

Symptoms of Deficiency: Retarded growth, poor appetite, and impaired smelling and taste sensation.

RDAs:		
	birth to 6 months	3 mg
	6 months to 1 year	5 mg
	1 to 10 years	10 mg

Unintended Effects: Commonly causes upset stomach and sometimes may even result in nausea and vomiting.

Drug and Food Interactions:

- Zinc reduces the absorption of tetracycline; both drugs should not be taken within two hours of each other.
- Food substances such as bran products, including brown bread, celery, lemon juice, coffee, hard-boiled eggs, and milk decrease the absorption of zinc.

Contraindication: Existing bleeding disorder of the gastrointestinal tract.

Special Notes:

- In children with a history of poor appetite, low growth percentiles, and sometimes erratic eating habits, marginal zinc deficiency should be suspected. However, rather than self-medicating with a zinc supplement, it is best to consult your health care provider first.
- Zinc deficiency may be associated with a type of skin disorder and delayed wound healing for which zinc treatment is indicated. However, do not give your child zinc supplement in an attempt to speed wound healing. Consult your health care provider if you suspect delayed wound healing in your child.
- The body's requirement for zinc is very small (see RDA), which is usually satisfied by dietary intake unless an individual is fed exclusively by vein, since parenteral feedings are free from any contaminants. That is when a special supplement may be needed.

Storage Instruction: Keep at room temperature.

CHAPTER 8

Medicines for Stomach and Intestinal Discomfort

This chapter briefly describes the physiology of the digestive system, the common illnesses affecting it, and the medicines that are used for their treatment. The purpose here is not to recommend specific medicines but rather to alert you about when to seek medical advice as well as to acquaint you with the most common ingredients in the nonprescription stomach and bowel remedies.

Physiology of the Digestive System

The digestive system (often called the GI, for gastrointestinal, system) comprises four regions: the esophagus, the stomach, the small intestine, and the large intestine. The esophagus is a long, hollow tube surrounded by layers of smooth muscle. It is connected to the stomach by a muscle called the pylorus. Once food has arrived in the stomach, the pylorus prevents it from being regurgitated back into the esophagus.

The stomach secretes acid to aid the breakdown of certain food substances and empties into the small intestine, which is the site for digestion and absorption. The lining of the intestine secretes a thick mucus to protect and lubricate the intestinal wall by neutralizing the acid and reducing contact with bacteria and irritants. The large intestine is responsible for absorption and storage. Any unabsorbed food residue, bacteria, and water are combined there to form fecal material. It also contains the nonharmful bacteria of the body, which contribute to the breakdown of waste products and the production of vitamin K and ammonia. These "helpful" bacteria are susceptible to changes in dietary habits, medicines, and gastrointestinal diseases. Complications may arise when the balance is upset.

The entire digestive system is controlled by a complex network of nerves, most of which are beyond the body's voluntary control. For instance, when a person feels tense or frightened, stimulation to intestinal movement and secretion slows down, which in turn also diminishes frequency of bowel movements. Everything returns to normal rhythm when the body relaxes.

Disorders such as indigestion, constipation, and diarrhea, which afflict adults, also occur in children, with different causes; so the treatment, likewise, may differ. The liver, the pancreas, and the biliary tract, which secretes bile into the small intestine for digestion, are also integral parts of the digestive system. However, disorders of these organs are not discussed in this chapter since they are not common in children. Instead, this chapter focuses on the common gastrointestinal abnormalities that may afflict your child in infancy, childhood, or adolescence.

Disorders of the Stomach and Intestines and Their Remedies

Disorder: Vomiting

In Infancy (Birth to Two Years)

Newborns and young infants may spit up milk as a result of excessive feeding, not letting gas out of the stomach by burping, or moving around after feedings. You can minimize this spitting by keeping your baby in a semi-sitting position following feedings and by frequent burping. Spitting up usually decreases by one year of age. If you have any reasons to suspect a more serious condition than those described here for spitting up, consult your health care provider for advice.

To distinguish spitting up from vomiting, you need to determine:

1. whether it is projectile vomiting or spitting up
2. whether the vomiting stops in twenty-four hours or lasts longer
3. its occurrence in relation to feeding and other associated symptoms such as fever, diarrhea, and upper respiratory symptoms
4. the color, consistency and odor of the vomitus

Normally, the vomitus from spitting up or regurgitation has the same color as the fluid fed to the child, a mucuslike consistency and a tolerable odor, unless the feeding consists of homogenized milk, in

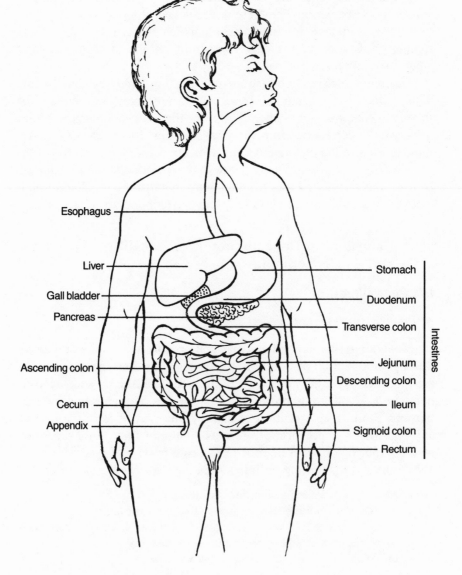

The anatomy of the digestive system.

which the butterfat may turn rancid and produce a strong odor. All of these can be differentiated from the yellowish and thick vomitus associated with an offensive odor.

To avoid choking on the vomitus during vomiting, hold your child's head downward to the side. After vomiting stops, do not give food or milk for several hours. Later offer small amounts of liquid (about a half-ounce), preferably clear fluids (those you can see through) such as water, tea, diluted apple juice, or popsicles, every fifteen to thirty minutes. If you choose to use commercial preparations of fluid and electrolytes (such as Pedialyte or Infalyte), consult the label for suggested doses for different age groups. These products are available in most grocery stores and pharmacies. As your child tolerates more, give up to two ounces of fluid each hour for twenty-four hours. If your child does not vomit the clear liquids, begin feeding other fluids, avoiding milk initially, and then gradually introduce bland solid foods, such as crackers and toast.

The major concern with vomiting in an infant is not only that the child is not absorbing nutrients from feeding but is also losing fluid and electrolytes from the body. You should seek medical attention if your child:

1. continues to vomit beyond twenty-four hours
2. cannot keep any fluid down
3. has a fever of 103° F or higher
4. appears restless or listless
5. diminishes urination frequency

In Children (Two to Twelve Years Old)

One of the reasons for a child in this age group to vomit is ingestion of foreign substances, which include plants, drugs, and household cleansing agents, such as soap or detergent. In that sense vomiting serves as a defense mechanism to eliminate undesirable substances from the body. During vomiting it is important to keep your child sitting up or resting on the side rather than lying flat. Although vomiting is the body's way of rejecting foreign objects, it can be harmful to induce vomiting for some types of ingestions, such as with corrosive or caustic substances, for example, bleach. Always contact your local Poison Control Center before inducing vomiting.

Eating contaminated food may also account for a sudden onset of vomiting. Symptoms usually begin within twenty-four hours after eating

118   *Nonprescription Medicines*

and may last several days, depending on the cause of the contamination. Associated symptoms include abdominal cramps, watery diarrhea, and fever. Should symptoms continue beyond twenty-four to forty-eight hours and if the child shows increasing difficulty in keeping fluid down, it is advisable to consult your health care provider for advice. Vomiting in general should be self-limiting, and treatment is primarily symptomatic, with fluid and electrolyte replacement and rest. You can introduce clear fluids, avoiding milk initially, and bland solid foods, such as crackers and toast, gradually as tolerated or as your child asks for food.

In Adolescents (Twelve Years and Older)

Self-induced vomiting (bulimia) should be suspected if it occurs regularly after meals. Some teenagers think that throwing up just eaten foods is one way to lose weight. This is not a healthy nor proper way to manage a weight problem and can lead to tragic consequences.

If a large weight loss occurs in a short period of time and no change in eating patterns is noticeable, you should consider looking into the cause of the drastic weight loss. You may not be aware that your adolescent induces vomiting after meals. Early recognition of this habit is imperative. Evidence has shown that if the self-induced vomiting continues beyond a certain length of time, it may be difficult to treat and health can deteriorate.

Chemical ingestion, either intentionally (e.g., as a suicidal gesture) or accidentally (e.g., siphoning gas or eating mushrooms for psychedelic effects) can occur among teenagers. Careful and sensitive questioning may provide clues to the cause behind it. With the exception of food poisoning, which usually gets better on its own, medical advice should be sought. This is especially so in the case of drug ingestion, since vomiting may be the beginning of some serious toxic effects.

Some systemic illnesses also produce vomiting as the first sign. Viral or bacterial meningitis (due to increased pressure inside the head), infectious hepatitis, gall bladder disorder, migraine headache, or even severe menstrual cramps can be associated with vomiting. However, these are usually accompanied by symptoms in addition to vomiting, so they should serve as a warning that medical attention is warranted.

Remedy: Antiemetic

DIMENHYDRINATE

Trade Names: Dimenhydrinate, Dimentabs, Dramamine, Eldodram, Marmine, Motion-Aid, Trav-Arex, Vertiban.

Dosage Forms: Liquid, tablet, suppository, injection.

Available in Generic Form: Yes.

Why Used: For the prevention and treatment of motion sickness.

How to Give: Read and follow the dosage and instructions for use on the label.

Time to Take Effect: Thirty minutes to one hour.

Unintended Effects: Drowsiness and dry mouth are common.

Drug and Food Interactions: Concurrent use of medicines with sedative properties enhances the drowsiness-inducing effect of this drug.

Contraindications:

- Previous allergy to this drug.
- Use with caution in children with severe asthma because of its drying effect.

Special Notes: Dimenhydrinate is not intended for the treatment of vomiting. As explained earlier in this chapter, vomiting due to benign causes is usually self-limiting and stops in one to two days; if not, the health care provider should be contacted for advice. This is especially important in children under five years because of dehydration and other potential complications.

Age Limitation: Not recommended for children under two years.

Storage Instruction: Keep at room temperature.

Disorder: Diarrhea

In Infancy (Birth to Two Years)

Diarrhea is the passage of loose, frequent, watery stools. The important factor is a change from the normal stool pattern. For the baby who usually has one stool every other day, three stools in one day may be diarrhea, whereas for another who normally has four stools daily, this is not.

Until the age of nine to twelve months a child's body is largely made up of fluid. Therefore profuse fluid loss from the body in the form of diarrheal stools can produce dehydration, shock, and in more severe cases, neurological symptoms such as lack of energy, irritability, convulsion, and coma. For this reason, if you are not sure of the degree of severity, if diarrhea lasts more than a day or two or is accompanied by vomiting, it is best to seek medical advice. To aid your health care provider in assessing the degree of dehydration, it is most helpful to know the child's weight prior to the onset of diarrhea. Also describe the number, frequency, consistency, odor, and color of the diarrhea, any other accompanying symptoms, and what you have been feeding your infant.

When the onset of diarrhea is sudden and accompanied by other viral symptoms like fever, running nose, or cough, it may be caused by a virus and stops with the other symptoms. Sudden, severe diarrhea is often caused by bacteria and needs to be treated quickly by a health care provider. Another possibility is that if your child is receiving an antibiotic for another illness such as an ear infection, the diarrhea may be the result of the antibiotic's destruction of the helpful bacteria in the bowel. In such an event, do not stop giving the medicine on your own. Consult whoever prescribed the medicine in the first place and seek alternative treatment.

Intolerance of the sugar that is present in all milk and milk products, including formulas, can manifest itself in diarrhea. Sugar malabsorption may be congenital or acquired following a bout of intestinal infection. In both cases a special formula needs to be substituted. It is best to consult your health care provider rather than attempting to switch formulas on your own. Second guessing may end up causing you unnecessary expense and be harmful to your child.

Gastrointestinal allergy to cow's milk proteins may also become apparent in early infancy. It is characterized by gradual onset of diarrhea and associated with vomiting and failure to gain weight. The degree of severity may range from relatively mild to severe diarrhea. Blood may even be passed with the stools. Other allergic symptoms such as dermatitis, asthma, and welts on the skin may also occur at the same time. Such a condition warrants medical attention and nutritional counseling, since multiple food allergies may also exist. Allergy to cow's milk protein is usually of limited duration, most children recovering by the age of two years.

The treatment of mild, nonspecific diarrhea is similar to that of vomiting: Begin with clear liquids, then gradually progress to other fluids, avoid milk initially, and then introduce solid foods. Constipating foods such as bananas, rice cereal, cooked carrots and squash are recommended for the first feedings following illness if your child has already started on solid foods of this kind.

However, if diarrhea is accompanied by bloody, black, or tarry stools or bloody vomiting, a sunken fontanel (soft spot on the head), a lack of tears when crying, a dry and sticky mouth, and less than three urinations per day, contact your health care provider immediately for treatment.

In Children (Two to Twelve Years Old)

Children in this age group can contract a nonspecific type of diarrhea in school or from other contact with children. Symptoms include various combinations and degrees of vomiting, diarrhea, nausea, abdominal cramps, headache, low-grade fever, loss of appetite, lack of energy, and muscle ache. Treatment for this type of diarrhea is the same as that for vomiting, fluid and electrolyte replacement. Fortunately, children recover on their own within a week or so. However, even with a nonspecific type of diarrhea, dehydration (excessive loss of body water) can still pose a problem. You should consult your health care provider if your child has any of the following symptoms:

- continues to have profuse, watery stools beyond twenty-four hours
- cannot keep any fluid down
- develops a fever of 103° F or higher
- appears restless or listless
- diminishes frequency of urinations per day

In Adolescents (Twelve Years and Older)

The most common reasons for acute diarrhea in adolescence are food poisoning, viral gastroenteritis, or drug-induced diarrhea, with antibiotics and laxatives being the most common offenders. A more serious but less common form of acute diarrhea among teenagers is inflammatory bowel disease. It constitutes a medical emergency because of the substantial loss of fluid, electrolytes, and even blood in the stool. Medical consultation is urgently needed.

Chronic diarrhea, on the other hand, characterized by small, frequent, watery stool associated with abdominal pain can be psychogenic or related to emotional stress. If this indeed is the case, some individuals can learn to live with the condition and it will be resolved over time; otherwise it is prudent to consult the health care provider to rule out other causes.

Remedy: Antidiarrheal

BISMUTH SUBSALICYLATE

Trade Names: Corrective Mixture, Pepto-Bismol.

Dosage Forms: Chewable tablet, suspension.

Available in Generic Form: Yes.

Why Used: An antidiarrheal agent with adsorbent property.

How to Give: Read and follow the dosage and instructions for use on the label.

Time to Take Effect: Thirty minutes to one hour.

Unintended Effect: This drug may at times result in constipation if it is over used.

Contraindication: Previous allergy to salicylate (aspirin).

Special Notes:
- May darken stool.
- Efficacy of this agent in coating or protecting the digestive tract as is often claimed is not proved.
- There is evidence of its effectiveness in the treatment and prevention of traveler's diarrhea.

Age Limitation: Not recommended for children under two years.

Storage Instruction: Keep at room temperature.

KAOLIN PECTIN

Trade Names: K-P, Kaolin w/Pectin, Kaomead, Kaopectate, Pargel.

Dosage Form: Suspension.

Available in Generic Form: Yes.

Why Used: It binds noxious materials in the intestine and solidifies or dries diarrheal stools.

How to Give: Read and follow the dosage and instructions for use on the label.

Time to Take Effect: One to four hours.

Unintended Effect: Unknown; safe to use.

Drug and Food Interactions: Avoid taking this drug with prescription medicines, since it may bind other medicines and render them ineffective.

Contraindication: Previous allergy to kaolin and pectin.

Special Note: Consult your health care provider if diarrhea continues beyond twenty-four hours, especially if your child is under five years.

Age Limitation: Consult manufacturer's recommendation on drug label or health care provider for use in children under five years.

Storage Instruction: Keep at room temperature.

OPIATES

Trade Names: Not as a single entity; present in combination products as opium powder, tincture of opium, and paregoric. Examples are Amogel PG, Corrective Mixture w/Paregoric, Diabismul, Dia-Zuel, Donnagel-PG, Infantol Pink, Kaodonna PG, Kaomead PG, Kapectolin PG, Kaodene #1, Kaodene #2, Kobac, Pabizol with Paregoric, Parelixir.

Dosage Forms: Tablet, liquid, suspension.

Available in Generic Form: Yes.

Why Used: Opiates are the most effective antidiarrheal agents; they slow down the propulsive movement of the intestine and stop bowel movements.

How to Give: Read and follow the dosage and instructions for use on the label.

Time to Take Effect: Within a few hours.

Unintended Effects:

- Drowsiness is common; often the drug preparation contains alcohol, which enhances the sedative effect, especially for a child.
- Persistent use may lead to addiction and complications affecting the intestinal wall.

Drug and Food Interactions: Any medicines with sedative properties will add to the drowsiness effect of the opiates.

Contraindications:

- Avoid using an opiate-containing drug to stop diarrhea of an infectious nature, since the toxic agents may be retained inside the intestine longer, thereby impeding recovery.
- Do not use in the presence of inflammatory bowel disease (colitis).
- Do not use if there is a history of allergy to any members of the opiate family (e.g., morphine, meperidine, codeine).

Special Notes: For occasional use in diarrhea of a benign nature, the opiates provide fast and safe relief.

Age Limitation: Consult manufacturer's recommendation on drug label or health care provider for use in children under two years.

Storage Instruction: Keep at room temperature.

Disorder: Constipation

In Infants (Birth to Two Years Old)

Hard, infrequent, and difficult-to-pass stools are occasional occurrences for most children. These may be streaked with a small amount of bright red blood, as the hard stool causes tears in the rectum. If your infant experiences this painful process and you are breast-feeding, add more fluid, fruits such as prunes, and bulk, such as whole grain breads and fresh, leafy vegetables to your own diet. Avoid constipating foods, such as cheese and bananas. A small amount of sugar (a half teaspoon for 4 ounces) can be added to the bottle-fed baby's formula for a few days to treat constipation. Or you can feed 1 to 2 teaspoons of dark corn syrup in 3 to 4 ounces of water once or twice daily for a few days. A glycerin suppository may be safe to use; however, it is a good idea to consult your health care provider before initiating treatment on your own.

In Children (Two to Twelve Years Old)

Constipation in childhood may be due to dietary habits, lack of time or discipline, drug intake (e.g., imipramine for bed-wetting has constipation as one of its unintended effects), anatomic defects, or psychological upsets including toilet training, birth of a sibling, moving to a new location, or the absence of a parent.

Normal bowel frequency ranges from one to three times a day to three to four times a week. It is necessary to know your child's normal bowel pattern in order to decide if constipation is present. Unless unusual symptoms set in, such as stomachache, pain in the anal area while stooling, or soiling, a dietary approach is advisable to treat constipation.

A low-fiber diet is conducive to constipation. Dietary fiber holds water; therefore, stools tend to be softer, bulkier, and pass through the colon more rapidly in a person with a reasonable amount of dietary fiber intake. Highly refined foods and low fiber content prolong intestinal transit time, thereby increasing the likelihood of constipation. As fluid is essential to aid the softening of the stool and its passage, fruit juices or other beverages should be offered as snacks. Whole grains, vegetables, fruits, and nuts have high fiber contents.

Resorting to laxatives without looking for the cause can be risky, for it may mask an underlying abnormality, thereby delaying treatment. Laxatives should be avoided in the presence of abdominal pain, because the sudden stimulation to the bowel may aggravate an existing disorder (for example, giving a laxative to a child with acute appendicitis is dangerous).

As you evaluate your child's bowel changes, look at the onset of constipation (gradual or sudden) and past bowel habits. Call your health care provider before using an enema or laxative on your own. Habitual use of these products is strongly discouraged, since increasing amounts are needed to produce results as the body's natural rhythms are suppressed.

In Adolescents (Twelve Years and Older)

Constipation in teenagers is also attributable to eating habits, life-style, or psychological reasons. Should your adolescent child develop persistent constipation, it would be ill advised to reach for the laxative right away, because life-long dependence on laxatives could follow. If you feel you need help to assist your child in resolving this problem, contact your health care provider for advice.

Eating habits not only contribute to bowel irregularities but can also result in indigestion. The best treatment is to correct a hasty style of eating or to select the types of food that "agree" with the stomach. Fatty and spicy foods are often the culprits. An occasional incidence of indigestion does not need medical treatment immediately. There are nonprescription products—the antacids—that can alleviate the heartburn sensation or stomach pain. When such a symptom becomes a regular occurrence and the stool begins to look very dark, a bleeding ulcer should be suspected and medical advice sought.

Remedy: Laxatives

BISACODYL

Trade Names: Bisacodyl, Bisco-Lax, Cenalax, Codylax, Deficol, Dulcolax, Fleet Bisacodyl, Laxadan Supules, Nuvac, SK-Bisacodyl, Theralax.

Dosage Forms: Enteric-coated tablet, suppository, enema.

Available in Generic Form: Yes.

Why Used: A stimulant laxative that works primarily on the colon and stimulates bowel movements.

How to Give: The tablet should not be crushed or taken with milk or antacid, which may dissolve the enteric coating and render the tablet irritating to the stomach. For a detailed discussion on how to give medicines by rectum, see Chapter 4.

Time to Take Effect: When applied rectally, action occurs within fifteen minutes to one hour; the tablet may take longer—within six to ten hours of administration.

Unintended Effect: Occasionally results in loose stools or diarrhea; generally considered a safe drug to use.

Drug and Food Interactions: Antacids and milk dissolve the enteric coating of the tablet and expose the inside of the tablet to the stomach, which can be discomforting.

Contraindications:

- Should not be given in the presence of stomachache or abdominal pain.
- Previous allergy to this drug.

Special Note: Avoid repetitive use of a laxative, since it disrupts normal bowel habits and dependence can result.

Age Limitation: Consult manufacturer's recommendation on drug label or health care provider for use in children under two years.

Storage Instruction: Keep the suppository in a cool place or refrigerated. Keep the other dosage forms at room temperature.

CASTOR OIL

Trade Names: Alphamul, Castor Oil, Emulsoil, Kellogg's Castor Oil, Neoloid, Purge.

Dosage Forms: Liquid, emulsion.

Available in Generic Form: Yes.

Why Used: Because of its potent purgative effect, it is usually used as a bowel preparation prior to diagnostic tests.

How to Give: Read and follow the dosage and instructions for use on the label.

Time to Take Effect: Two to six hours.

Unintended Effects:

- Potentially causes damage to the absorptive organs of the intestinal wall upon repeated use.
- Also causes the body to lose both water and electrolytes.

Drug and Food Interaction: No significant interaction reported.

Contraindications:

- Should not be used in the presence of stomachache or abdominal pain.
- Previous allergy to this drug.

Special Note: Avoid repetitive use of a laxative, since it disrupts normal bowel habits and dependence on the drug can result.

Age Limitation: Consult manufacturer's recommendation on drug label or health care provider for use in children under two years.

Storage Instruction: Keep at room temperature.

DSS (DIOCTYL SODIUM SULFOSUCCINATE)

Trade Names: Afko-Lube, Bu-Lax 100, Colace, Coloctyl, Comfolax, Disonate, Diosuccin, Dio-Sul, Docusate Sodium, DSS, Doxinate, Duosol, Modane Soft, Dolatoc, Regutol, Stulex.

Dosage Forms: Capsule, tablet, liquid, syrup, enema.

Available in Generic Form: Yes.

Why Used: A lubricant laxative that acts like a detergent, retaining water in the intestine and facilitating the mixing of fatty and watery substances, thereby softening the stool and aiding its evacuation.

How to Give: Read and follow the dosage and instructions for use on the label.

Time to Take Effect: Twelve to seventy-two hours.

Unintended Effect: No significant side effects reported.

Drug and Food Interactions: Enhances the absorption of mineral oil through the intestine into the body when used together, and an inflammatory response may result.

Contraindications:

- Use with caution in the presence of stomachache or abdominal pain.
- Previous allergy to this drug.

Special Notes:

- This is basically a stool softener that works best before the stool hardens and becomes impacted, which is indicated by straining during a bowel movement.
- Avoid repetitive use of a laxative, since it disrupts normal bowel habits and dependence on the drug can result.

Age Limitation: Consult manufacturer's recommendation on drug label or health care provider for use in children under two years.

Storage Instruction: Keep in a cool, dry place or refrigerated, otherwise the capsules may stick together. Keep the liquid at room temperature and the mouth of the bottle clean, otherwise the cap may get stuck to the bottle.

GLYCERIN

Trade Names: Fleet Babylax, Glycerin.

Dosage Forms: Liquid for rectal use, suppository.

Available in Generic Form: Yes.

Why Used: It exerts pressure inside the intestine to stimulate bowel movements and pulls water into the colon to soften stool.

How to Give: Read and follow the dosage and instructions for use on the label. For a detailed discussion on how to give medicines by rectum, see Chapter 4.

Time to Take Effect: Fifteen minutes to one hour.

Unintended Effect: Occasionally, discomfort to the rectum; generally considered a safe drug to use.

Drug and Food Interaction: No significant interaction reported.

Contraindications:

- Should not be given in the presence of stomachache or abdominal pain.
- Previous allergy to this drug.

Special Notes:

- There is an oral liquid preparation available (glycerol), but it is not used as a laxative.
- Avoid repetitive use of a laxative, since it disrupts normal bowel habits and dependence on the drug can result.

Age Limitation: Can be used in children under two years.

Storage Instruction: Keep refrigerated.

MAGNESIUM CITRATE

Trade Names: Citrate of Magnesia, Citroma, Citro-Nesia.

Dosage Form: Liquid.

Available in Generic Form: Yes.

Why Used: A saline laxative that draws fluid into the intestine and induces bowel movements.

How to Give: Read and follow the dosage and instructions for use on the label.

Time to Take Effect: Thirty minutes to three hours.

Unintended Effect: Rarely causes electrolyte imbalance; generally considered a safe drug to use.

Drug and Food Interaction: No significant interaction reported.

Contraindications:

- Should be avoided in the presence of kidney disease.
- Should be avoided in the presence of stomachache or abdominal pain.

Special Notes:

- The bottle should be chilled for palatability.
- It is carbonated; once the bottle is opened, it may not be able to be recapped without losing carbonation.

Age Limitation: Consult manufacturer's recommendation on drug label or health care provider for use in children under two years.

Storage Instruction: Keep refrigerated.

MAGNESIUM HYDROXIDE

Trade Name: Milk of Magnesia.

Dosage Form: Suspension.

Available in Generic Form: Yes.

Why Used: A saline laxative that draws fluid into the intestine and induces bowel movements.

How Used: Read and follow the dosage and instructions for use on the label.

Time to Take Effect: Thirty minutes to three hours.

Unintended Effect: Loose stools.

Drug and Food Interaction: No significant interaction reported.

Contraindications:

- Should be avoided in the presence of kidney disease.
- Should be avoided in the presence of stomachache or abdominal pain.

Special Notes:

- It is often used in combination with other ingredients in antacid preparations, although its acid neutralizing action is not related to its laxative property.
- Avoid repetitive use of a laxative since it disrupts normal bowel habits and dependence on the drug can result.

Age Limitation: Consult manufacturer's recommendation on drug label or health care provider for use in children under two years.

Storage Instruction: Keep at room temperature.

MINERAL OIL

Trade Names: Agoral Plain, Mineral Oil, Neo-Cultol, Nujol, Kondremul Plain, Petrogalar Plain, Zymenol.

Dosage Forms: Liquid, emulsion, jelly, suspension.

Available in Generic Form: Yes.

Why Used: Lubricates the intestinal tract and softens fecal material for easy evacuation.

How to Give: Read and follow the dosage and instructions for use on the label. Single doses should be given at bedtime or at least several hours after a meal.

Time to Take Effect: Six to eight hours.

Unintended Effects:

- Absorption of mineral oil into the body may elicit an inflammatory response inside the intestine; the drug is ordinarily not absorbed through the intestinal wall.
- Chronic use may result in leakage through the anus, causing skin irritation.
- Aspiration of mineral oil into the airway produces an inflammatory response in the lungs (i.e., pneumonitis).

Drug and Food Interactions:

- Mineral oil impairs the absorption of vitamins A, D, E, and K; thus they should not be taken together. For this reason mineral oil should not be used on a long-term basis.
- DSS enhances the absorption of mineral oil; these should not be taken together.

Contraindications:

- Should not be used in the presence of stomachache or abdominal pain.
- Avoid using this drug in the presence of unconsciousness or in someone without gag reflex or with difficulty in swallowing. These conditions may enhance the likelihood of aspiration.
- Previous allergy to this drug.

Special Notes:

- Despite its safety and effectiveness, this drug should not be used persistently because of the potential undesirable effects.
- Avoid repetitive use of a laxative since it disrupts normal bowel habits and dependence on the drug can result.

Age Limitation: The oral form is not recommended for children under five years.

Storage Instruction: Keep at room temperature.

PHENOLPHTHALEIN

Trade Names: Alophen Pills, Correctol, Evac-U-Lax, Ex-Lax, Feen-a-Mint Gum, Feen-a-Mint, Phenolax, Prulet.

Dosage Forms: Chewable and regular tablet, liquid, wafer.

Available in Generic Form: Yes.

Why Used: Causes local irritation of the lining of the intestinal wall and increases the propulsive activity of the intestine. It may also prevent the absorption of water and electrolytes from the intestine into the body, thus promoting evacuation of the bowel.

How to Give: Read and follow the dosage and instructions for use on the label.

Time to Take Effect: Six to eight hours.

Drug and Food Interaction: No significant interaction reported.

Unintended Effect:

- May produce severe diarrhea, resulting in electrolyte imbalance, especially in children under five years.
- Some of the tablets or wafers contain a dye that has been known to be sensitizing—it can result in skin reactions such as hives, rash, and itchiness.

Contraindications:

- Previous allergy to this drug or the dye contained in the tablet.
- Should not be used in the presence of stomachache or abdominal pain.

Special Notes:

- May turn urine red-violet, red-brown, pink-red or yellow-brown, depending on the pH of the urine.
- As a chocolate-flavored bar, youngsters may mistake it for candy; severe diarrhea with excessive loss of fluid and electrolytes can result. Thus when used by a family member, it should be kept out of reach of young children.
- Avoid repetitive use of a laxative since it disrupts normal bowel habits and dependence on the drug can result.

Age Limitation: Not recommended for children under two years.

Storage Instruction: Keep at room temperature.

PHOSPHOSODA

Trade Names: Phospho-Soda, Sal-Hepatica.

Dosage Forms: Powder, liquid, enema (regular and pediatric in size, low-sodium and regular in content).

Available in Generic Form: Yes.

Why Used: A saline laxative that draws fluid into the intestine and induces bowel movements.

How to Give: Read and follow the dosage and instructions for use on the label. For a detailed discussion of how to give medicines by rectum, see Chapter 4.

Time to Take Effect: One to four hours.

Unintended Effect: May produce electrolyte imbalance in a child under six years.

Drug and Food Interaction: No significant interaction reported.

Contraindications:

- Should not be used in the presence of severe heart or kidney disease.
- Should not be used in the presence of stomachache or abdominal pain.

Special Note: Avoid repetitive use of a laxative since it disrupts normal bowel habits and dependence on the drug can result.

Age Limitation: Not recommended for children under six years.

Storage Instruction: Keep at room temperature.

PSYLLIUM SEED

Trade Names: Hydrocil, L. A. Formula, Metamucil, Modane Bulk, Mucilose, Regacilium, Reguloid, Syllact, Siblin, V-Lax.

Dosage Forms: Granules, effervescent and regular powder.

Available in Generic Form: Yes.

Why Used: A bulk-forming laxative that forms a lubricating gel inside the intestine and facilitates the passage of stools.

How to Give: Read and follow the dosage and instructions on the label. This medicine should be mixed with fluid for administration or constipation results.

Time to Take Effect: Twelve hours to three days.

Unintended Effect: Intestinal obstruction, when taken in the dry form.

Drug and Food Interactions: May bind other medicines and inhibit their absorption.

Contraindications:

- Should not be used in the presence of stomachache, abdominal pain, or intestinal obstruction.
- Previous allergy to this drug or other members of the plantain family.

Special Notes:

- Be sure to administer this drug with a large amount of fluid (6 to 8 ounces).
- Should be mixed with water or juice immediately prior to administration; if allowed to sit, the solution will thicken or gel.
- It is sometimes used in the management of irritable bowel syndrome and is therefore used on a long-term basis.

Age Limitation: Consult manufacturer's recommendation on drug label or health care provider for use in children under two years.

Storage Instruction: Keep at room temperature.

SENNA EXTRACT

Trade Names: Black-Draught, Casafru, Senokot, X-Prep.

Dosage Forms: Granules, tablet, powder, liquid, syrup, suppository.

Available in Generic Form: Yes.

Why Used: Stimulates bowel movement of the intestine by local irritation of the lining of the intestinal wall.

How to Give: Read and follow the dosage and instructions for use on the label.

Time to Take Effect: Eight to twelve hours.

Drug and Food Interaction: No significant interaction reported.

Unintended Effects:

- Occasionally causes stomach discomfort.
- May turn urine red-violet, red-brown, pink-red, or yellow-brown, depending on pH of the urine.

Contraindications:

- Should not be used in the presence of stomachache or abdominal pain.
- Previous allergy to this drug or other members of the anthraquinone family.

Special Notes: None.

Age Limitation: Consult manufacturer's recommendation on drug label or health care provider for use in children under two years.

Storage Instruction: Keep at room temperature. Keep the mouth of the bottle containing the syrup clean, otherwise the cap may get stuck.

Remedies for Occasional Stomach Discomfort

ANTACIDS

Trade Names: Alkets, Aludrox, A-M-T, Camalox, Creamalin, Delcid, Di Gel, Estomul, Estomul-M, Eugel, Flacid, Gaviscon, Gaviscon-2, Gelusil, Kolantyl, Kudrox, Magnatril, Magnagel, Maalox #1, Maalox #2, Maalox Plus, Mylanta, Mylanta II, Noralac, Neutracomp, Neutralox, Riopan Plus, Rolaids, Simaal Gel, Simeco, Silain-Gel, Tritralac, Trisogel, Trialka, Win-Gel.

Dosage Forms: Chewable tablet, capsule, suspension.

Available in Generic Form: Yes.

Why Used: For neutralization of excessive secretion of stomach acid and digestive enzyme (pepsin) and for relief of occasional stomach discomfort from sour stomach, acid indigestion, or heartburn.

Here are the different neutralizing ingredients in antacids and their effectiveness:

1. Aluminum hydroxide (trade names: Alucap, Aluminum Hydroxide Gel, U.S.P., AlternaGEL, Alu-Tab, Amphojel, Dialume).

   Available singly or in combination in several brands of antacids. When used alone it is a weak acid neutralizer. The main disadvantage of this drug is its constipating effect. Chronic use (over weeks and months) of this drug depletes the body of phosphate and increases aluminum to an undesirably high level. Low phosphate produces fatigue, loss of appetite, and muscle weakness, and high aluminum level is manifested in degenerative neurological symptoms (e.g., difficulty in concentrating, forgetfulness, disorientation, or even hallucination).

2. Calcium carbonate (trade names: Alka-2, Amitone, Calcium Carbonate, Chooz, Dicarbosil, Equilet, Mallamint, P.H. Tabs, Tums).

   This is a potent and effective antacid that can induce an opposite reaction in the stomach—the increased production of acid. However, for occasional use this does not need to be a concern. The main disadvantage of using calcium alone as an antacid is its constipating effect. Absorption of calcium from this drug into the body depends on the dose taken. Usually constipation sets in before a dangerously high level of calcium occurs.

3. Magnesium hydroxide (trade name: Milk of Magnesia, Mint-o-mag).

   Similar to aluminum hydroxide, magnesium hydroxide is available singly or in combination with other ingredients in several brands of antacid. The main disadvantage of using this drug alone is that it causes loose stools or diarrhea. Thus it is better taken in combination with aluminum hydroxide. This is an effective antacid except for children with kidney disease, in which case it should be avoided altogether. Magaldrate (Riopan) is a chemical entity of aluminum and magnesium hydroxide. It has a low sodium content and is marketed for this very purpose.

4. Sodium bicarbonate (trade names: Bell/ans, Sodium Bicarbonate, Soda-Mint).

   Sodium bicarbonate is a potent and effective antacid. Chronic use of this drug is inadvisable, because sodium is absorbed into the body and for children with heart or kidney disease that can be hazardous. In addition, this drug is so potent that it can alter the pH balance in blood as well, which may result in undesirable effects. The effervescence of the tablet releases gas and causes stomach distention, which may further

stimulate acid secretion. For occasional fast relief of indigestion, this drug is safe to use, but it is best avoided for long-term administration.
5. Simethicone (trade name: Mylicon).

Simethicone is not an antacid since it does not have any neutralizing power, but it is claimed to break up gas bubbles in the stomach, thereby alleviating the associated discomfort. The truth of this claim is yet to be proved, but it is a relatively safe drug to use.

How to Give: For occasional stomach discomfort, select either the tablet or the suspension form of an antacid of your choice. The tablet should be chewed before swallowing. Read and follow the dosage and instructions for use on the label.

Time to Take Effect: Usually within thirty minutes.

Unintended Effects:

• The magnesium component of antacids may cause loose stools or diarrhea.
• The aluminum component of antacids may cause constipation.
• Some antacids contain a substantial amount of sodium, which may not be tolerated in the presence of heart or kidney disease.

Drug and Food Interactions: Avoid taking antacids with tetracycline and iron supplement, because antacids reduce their absorption.

Contraindications:

• Sodium-containing antacids should be avoided in the presence of kidney and heart disease.
• Magnesium-containing antacids should be avoided in the presence of kidney disease.
• Previous allergy to any ingredients in the antacid.

Special Notes:

• The potency of an antacid (its ability to give relief) is measured by its acid-neutralizing capacity. There is an optimal range of acidity for pepsin (a digestive enzyme) to function in the breaking down of food particles. A drastic reduction of acidity can cause the opposite effect—stimulation of acid secretion. Therefore it is advisable to select a product that does not overcompensate and to follow the recommended instructions for use. Consult a pharmacist on the selection of a brand that is best suited for your child's need.
• Flavor is an important consideration in the selection of an antacid, especially if your child has a special preference. Several of the existing products have peppermint and fruit flavor to enhance consumer accep-

tance. For an occasional use, they are comparable in effectiveness. However, they should still be treated as medicines but not candies and should be taken with discretion and care. Dosage and instructions for use are on the label or in the individual package.

Age Limitation: Consult manufacturer's recommendation on drug label or health care provider for use in children under two years.

Storage Instruction: Keep at room temperature.

Miscellaneous

ACTIVATED CHARCOAL

Trade Names: Activated Charcoal U.S.P., Charcodote, Res-Q.

Drug Class: Antidote, a drug used in the treatment of poisoning.

Dosage Forms: Powder, tablet.

Available in Generic Form: Yes.

Why Used: Because of its massive surface area for adsorption, it is useful in binding toxic substances to aid in their removal from the body.

How to Give: Usually used in conjunction with syrup of ipecac in the treatment of poisoning or ingestion of toxic substances. Charcoal is a black powder and unpleasant to take, so flavoring agents can be added such as ice cream, chocolate syrup, cocoa powder, jam, or jelly. Dosage and instructions for use should be obtained from a Poison Control Center or a health professional.

Unintended Effect: Constipation.

Drug and Food Interaction: Activated charcoal diminishes the action of ipecac when both drugs are taken at the same time. Always give the syrup of ipecac first before giving activated charcoal.

Contraindication: Do not give this medicine without consulting a Poison Control Center or a health professional.

Special Notes:

- Due to its constipating effect, it is customary practice to give a laxative following the administration of this drug. An additional purpose of the laxative is to help purge the toxic substances from the body.

- Activated charcoal is sold without a prescription in a 1-ounce bottle in pharmacies and convenience stores. It is a handy first aid agent to keep on hand in your home. Purchase the powder rather than the tablet, since the latter's adsorptive power is considerably less because of the smaller surface area.
- Burned toast does not have the pharmacologic properties of activated charcoal; the latter's enormous surface area has been demonstrated to be helpful in binding certain toxic substances.
- If syrup of ipecac is used to induce vomiting, it should be given prior to activated charcoal. Only after vomiting has occurred should charcoal be given, since it impairs ipecac's ability to stimulate vomiting.
- Since this drug is not equally effective against all poisons, consult the health care provider or Poison Control Center for advice prior to administering this drug at home.

Age Limitation: Consult Poison Control Center or health care provider before using this drug.

Storage Instruction: Keep at room temperature and in a dry place. Charcoal may absorb moisture in the air if the lid of the bottle is not on tightly.

SYRUP OF IPECAC

Trade Name: Syrup of Ipecac U.S.P.

Dosage Form: Syrup.

Available in Generic Form: Yes.

Why Used: To induce vomiting.

How to Give: Always consult a Poison Control Center or your health care provider before administering this drug. In general the doses are as follows:

Weight	Dose
25 lbs and under	1 tablespoon
Over 25 lbs	1 to 2 tablespoons

Time to Take Effect: Twenty to thirty minutes.

Unintended Effect: Rarely causes continuous vomiting (over two hours).

Drug and Food Interaction: Milk diminishes the action of ipecac. Always give clear fluids only with the syrup of ipecac.

Contraindications:

- Should not be used in an unconscious, sleepy, or convulsing child.
- Should not be used when a corrosive or caustic substance is ingested.

Special Notes:

- This is the most widely used emetic and can be purchased without a prescription. However, prior to using this drug, be sure to consult a Poison Control Center or a health professional, because vomiting is not called for in every instance of ingestion, especially with chemicals such as bleach, acid, and certain petroleum products.
- If adequate fluid is taken (6 to 8 ounces), vomiting should begin within twenty to thirty minutes of drug administration and a second dose is usually not needed. However, if vomiting does not occur within that time after plenty of fluid, contact the Poison Control Center again for further instructions before giving a second dose.
- Always give clear liquid with this drug; milk may diminish its effectiveness.
- There is no need to hold the child still after administering the drug, but an upright position rather than lying down is imperative once vomiting begins.
- Syrup of Ipecac is a safe and effective first-aid agent; it is a good idea to keep a bottle on hand for emergency use.

Age Limitation: Consult Poison Control Center or health care provider before using this drug.

Storage Instruction: Keep at room temperature.

CHAPTER 9

Medicines for Breathing Difficulties

Few things are more frightening to a parent than for a child to have difficulty breathing. An understanding of how the respiratory system works helps parents cope with this situation. This chapter discusses the disorders that impair breathing in different age groups, and medicines for their treatment. Congenital defects resulting in chronic breathing problems or respiratory failure are beyond the scope of this book.

Physiology of Breathing

The respiratory system comprises several anatomical structures: the nose, the nasal cavities, the pharynx (the throat), the trachea, the bronchiole tree, and the lungs. Inside the nose is a continuous lining of mucous membrane with a dense supply of blood vessels, nerves, mucus glands, and fine, hairlike elements known as cilia. The rich vascular bed and the mucous glands warm and humidify the inhaled air before it reaches the lungs. Simultaneously, the nasal secretions also have a protective role, for they contain digestive enzymes and antibodies to fight bacteria and viruses. In addition, the constant wavelike movement of the cilia helps propel any foreign particles toward the pharynx, where they are either expelled through the mouth or swallowed into the esophagus.

The mucous membrane is, however, subject to infection and inflammation. When this happens, it becomes swollen and hypersecretory, which results in nasal congestion. Medications taken orally or applied topically can reduce the swelling and dry the secretion by means of their pharmacological action on the nerves and blood vessels.

The pharynx connects the upper respiratory organs to the lower units. It divides into the esophagus and the trachea, which is why we "breathe" through the mouth when the nose loses its function. The trachea branches into two bronchi, each supplying air to one lung. Each bronchus further divides into bronchioles, which ultimately end in small air sacs known as alveoli. Gaseous exchange occurs between the thin surface of the alveoli and the tiny blood vessels (the capillaries) that lie adjacent to the alveoli. The lower respiratory units are, like the nose,

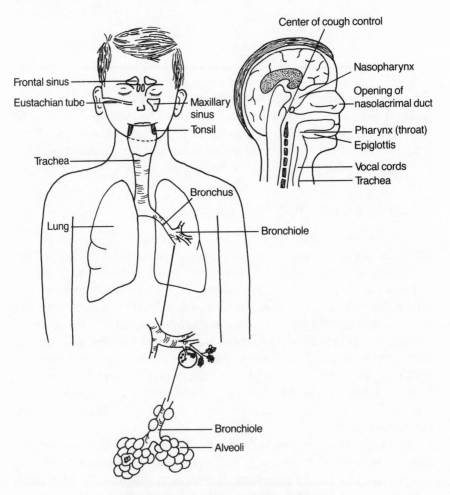

The anatomy of the breathing passages.

lined by a ciliated lining of mucous membrane and have a rich supply of mucous glands, blood vessels, and nerve tissues. The trachea, bronchi, and bronchioles are encircled by smooth muscle, which contracts and dilates in response to pharmacologic agents, chemicals, or foreign substances present in the body (i.e., allergens). The lungs are light, spongy, and enclosed by a double-walled structure known as the pleura. The interior of the pleura is normally airtight.

The secondary respiratory organs are the rib cage, its connective tissues, and the diaphragm, which lies between the thoracic cavity and the abdomen. The diaphragm is a dome-shape structure at rest, extending upward into the thoracic cavity. When we inhale, the diaphragm flattens, the chest wall pushes outward, and the thoracic cavity becomes enlarged and the pressure within the cavity lessens, thereby allowing air to enter. When we exhale, the diaphragm relaxes, resuming its usual dome shape. The rest of the secondary respiratory organs also relax, providing sufficient pressure inside the chest wall to produce exhalation.

Disorders of the Respiratory Tract

Allergic Rhinitis

Allergic rhinitis is a condition characterized by a runny nose, nasal stuffiness, and watery mucus discharge. These symptoms may occur at specific seasons or year-round. In addition to the nasal symptoms, the child may also complain of itching and watering in both eyes or other skin irritation, such as eczema. Frequently there is a strong family history of allergy.

For the relief of mild symptoms, you may choose to select a nonprescription decongestant either in a nosedrop or an oral form, plus an antihistamine such as brompheniramine or chlorpheniramine. However, if symptoms worsen or if no relief is offered by the over-the-counter remedy, you should contact your health care provider for advice.

Asthma

Asthma is characterized by airway obstruction that results from spasm of the smooth muscle, called bronchoconstriction, of the bronchioles, swelling and inflammation of the mucous membrane lining the airways, and hypersecretion of the cells in the bronchial tree. All these are triggered by elevated levels of biological substances such as histamines, slow-releasing substances in the body that are secreted in response to allergens. The diameter of the airways can narrow and widen depending on how the body's nervous and immune systems respond. The diameter of the airways affects the amount of air allowed into the lungs. Medicines for asthma relax and dilate the bronchial smooth muscle and counteract the effects of substances that produce bronchoconstriction.

While asthma may begin at any age, the majority of asthmatic children experience their first symptoms before four to five years. A family history of hay fever or other types of allergies is strongly suggestive of the illness. Some of these children grow out of their illness when they reach puberty. Recurrent episodes of coughing and wheezing, especially if they are induced by exercise, should lead the parent to suspect a tendency toward asthma.

Children are affected to various degrees. If your child has an attack once a week or less and is essentially free of any respiratory symptoms the rest of the time, then he or she may not need continuous drug therapy. A child who coughs and wheezes frequently even without any exacerbation (e.g., exercise or a cold) or who loses sleep at night needs continuous treatment with a bronchodilator. Evaluation by the health care provider is necessary to determine the degree of severity and the attendant treatment.

A child suspected to have asthma needs a careful examination to identify the allergens and events associated with an asthmatic attack. Parents and the health care provider can determine if continuous drug therapy is needed. The most effective agents to date for treating asthma are available by prescription only. Most nonprescription asthma products contain a combination of ingredients, some of which are of questionable value.

Bronchiolitis

Bronchiolitis is an inflammatory obstruction of the small airways. It occurs primarily between birth and two years, with a peak incidence at about six months and the highest frequency in winter and early spring. It is a viral illness that may begin with an older family member. Infants are affected more seriously by the presence of swelling and accumulation of mucus because of their relatively small bronchial trees. The initial symptoms include nasal discharge, sneezing, fever, and diminished appetite. Breathing difficulty gradually develops, which is accompanied by wheezing, cough, and irritability. Feeding may be difficult, since the rapid rate of breathing may not allow time for sucking and swallowing. The most critical phase is during the first two to three days after the onset of cough and shortness of breath. Because the child who is likely to contract this illness is usually under two years old, no over-the-counter medicines are available for relief of symptoms. The degree of breathing difficulty in the child should help parents decide whether to seek medical advice.

Bronchitis

Bronchitis is inflammation of the bronchi and is more common in children over six years old. It can be bacterial as well as viral in origin and is usually preceded by a viral upper respiratory infection such as a cold. The child has a frequent, dry, hacking, and unproductive cough for three to four days. As the illness progresses, whistling sounds are noticed during respiration, associated with occasional shortness of breath. Gradually the cough turns productive and the sputum changes from clear to thick and yellow. An expectorant at this time would be appropriate to facilitate the removal of sputum from the respiratory tract.

The child may also have a low-grade fever (101° F or under), runny nose, and inflammation of the eyes. The entire episode may last from one to three weeks, and complications are few. Most children recover without any specific treatment. If coughing interferes with sleep, a dose of antitussive (a drug used to stop coughing) at bedtime is appropriate. Antihistamines dry secretions and may aggravate the condition, so they are best avoided. Depending on the severity of the symptoms and the level of your child's discomfort, you should contact your health care provider for advice.

Common Cold

The common cold is by far the most usual cause of a stuffy or runny nose. The illness is viral in origin, and there is no specific therapy to shorten or cure a cold. Antibiotics have no role in its treatment unless there is a secondary bacterial infection; this is more common in children than in adults. There also seems to be a seasonal pattern to the common cold, the peaks occurring typically in the fall about the time school begins, in mid-winter, and in spring toward the end of April.

Children get infected in nursery or grade school or through contacts with siblings or other family members. Their symptoms also appear to be more severe than those of adults.

Cold symptoms, such as fever, headache, fatigue, nasal discharge, and decreased appetite, may be the early symptoms of other communicable diseases, namely influenza or flu, which is caused by a more virulent type of virus; measles; and pertussis. In these cases medical attention is needed. In addition, a common cold may be complicated by middle-ear infection, especially in the young child, or infection of other parts of the respiratory tract. The clue to these complications is a fever above 101° F that recurs after the most severe symptoms of a cold have seemingly subsided, or when the child starts complaining of pain in the ear or pulling at it or showing breathing difficulty.

Remedies for a common cold are primarily rest and fluid intake. Should your child appear not to have an appetite, this is not the time to force nourishment, but the intake of fluids should be encouraged frequently. Nasal congestion can be relieved with an oral decongestant or a topical nosedrop. For the young infant who is dependent on nose-breathing, a congested nose may lead to respiratory distress and interfere with feeding and sleeping. Most nonprescription medicated nosedrops are not recommended for use in children under two. A normal saline solution, which can be purchased without a prescription, can be used to dilute the mucus inside the nasal cavities, and a bulb syringe can then be used to suction out the mucus (see Appendix 3). In addition, a humidified environment such as that provided by a vaporizer also aids in the relief of breathing difficulty.

For the child older than two years of age, an assortment of medicated decongestant nosedrops can be purchased. Some take effect rapidly but are short-acting, requiring frequent administration. Overuse of a nosedrop or spray has been known to cause increased congestion, compounding the problem it was meant to treat and prolonging the discomfort. It is advisable, therefore, to select a longer-acting drug for use over a limited time, such as four to five days. Should the symptoms continue, it can be used again. The judicious use of this type of medicine is important, since it otherwise can provide more harm than benefit. If your child is too young to use a nose spray, select a dropper bottle and administer it yourself (see Chapter 4 on giving medications by nose).

Most topical nosedrops act by shrinking the swelling of the mucosal tissue, constricting the blood vessels and secretory glands to reduce mucus. Oral decongestants are not as effective as some of the topical agents for relief of breathing difficulty, and since some of them are combined with antihistamines, they are best avoided. Antihistamines dry the mucous membrane, rendering the pharynx susceptible to irritation, and may even produce a dry, sore throat. They also cause drowsiness and dull alertness, interfering with many activities.

An antitussive is also not necessary even if the child coughs occasionally. Depressing the cough reflex with a drug may increase the chance of inhaling into the lungs material secreted from the nasal cavities and the pharynx. A mild antitussive may be helpful at night so that a cough does not interfere with your child's sleep.

Teenagers who may self-medicate need to be cautioned about the overuse of nosedrops or nasal spray. They should be told of the disadvantage of taking a combination of a decongestant and an antihistamine especially because of the latter's sedative effect.

Croup

Croup is a mild form of respiratory distress syndrome common in children between three months to five years, especially during the winter months. It is a viral illness that produces inflammation of the vocal cords extending to the trachea. The preliminary manifestations are one to two days of upper respiratory symptoms characterized by a mild, brassy cough with an intermittent harsh, low-pitched inspiratory sound, called stridor, and a hoarse voice. Fever is often present. Breathing difficulty ranges from mild to severe, but the breathing rate increases and so does the pulse. Sucking in of the chest and abdominal muscles is evident, indicating some real effort in breathing. The child typically prefers to sit up in bed or be held upright; agitation and crying aggravate the symptoms. Depending on the parents' ability to manage the child's symptoms, the extent of the child's breathing difficulty, and his or her response to home treatment, the health care provider should be contacted for advice.

The most common method used to ease breathing difficulty is a cool vaporizer or steam from a hot shower or bath in a closed bathroom. Breathing difficulty may be relieved within minutes.

If the child's breathing appears slow and labored, the extremities are cold, a bluish-gray tinge appears on the lips and face, and the child looks pale and confused, immediate medical attention is necessary. These are indicative of the lack of oxygen in the body.

Drug Ingestion

Accidental ingestion of a large dose of sedatives or some nonprescription antihistamines, which are commonly found in cold remedies, causes respiratory depression. Maintaining an open airway is imperative if your child is having breathing difficulty. Then it is important to find out if it is drug-related. Getting intoxicated by alcohol after ingesting an excessive dose of a depressant would produce slow and shallow breathing. It is dangerous to induce vomiting in such a condition, since the child could choke on the vomitus, resulting in aspiration pneumonia. Medical attention is definitely warranted. You should contact a Poison Control Center or your health care provider for advice immediately.

Epiglottitis

Epiglottitis is a bacterial infection of the epiglottis, which is located in the back of the throat. It has the highest incidence among two- to six-year-olds. The onset is abrupt, and the disease progresses rapidly within hours. It is not necessarily preceded by any respiratory illness, although a child may have a fever and sore throat. Soon after these symptoms, swallowing becomes difficult and painful, so the child drools and is irritable and restless. The voice is muffled but not hoarse. Breathing difficulty is apparent and gets progressively worse. The child typically insists on sitting upright or leaning slightly forward with his or her neck extended, mouth open, and chin jutting out to allow the widest airway opening in the tracheal region. In general, the child looks very sick. The condition requires prompt medical attention, and no attempt should be made to examine the throat or give any medicine by mouth for relief. Contact the health care provider or an emergency room for advice and assistance immediately.

Foreign Body

It is not unusual for children to place any number of small objects in the nose or throat. Peanuts, crayons, beads, paper, marbles, or small toys are among the objects they may choose. When only the nose is affected, initial symptoms are sneezing, mild pain, and local obstruction. The irritation caused by the foreign object results in swelling of the mucous membrane. Depending on the property of the foreign body, it may grow in size as it absorbs water, thus increasing the obstruction and discomfort associated with it. A clue to the possible presence of a foreign body in the nose is when obstruction occurs only on one side. Careful questioning of the young child instead of a punitive approach may reveal what the child placed in his or her nose. If presence of a foreign body is suspected, removal should be done promptly and warrants an office visit to a health care provider if the object is not clearly visible and easily removable by you. Removal aside, there are no medicines for treatment.

When a foreign object is stuck in the trachea, the child usually gags, chokes, or coughs at first and goes on to develop shortness of breath. If the child shows signs of suffocation immediately after the swallowing, called aspiration, try to keep the airway open, administer aid for airway obstruction, and call for emergency help. Breathing difficulty may occur immediately after the swallowing or days later, as swelling develops around the foreign object or as it becomes lodged in a more obstructive position. If you do not witness the acute episode, symptoms that are to occur later, such as an occasional cough or slight wheezing, may not be easily recognized by you as symptoms of a foreign body in the respiratory tract. Sometimes these symptoms may progress to pneumonia or asthma. Contact your health care provider if foreign body aspiration is suspected.

Sinusitis

If, following the acute phase of a cold, congestion continues, with the additional discomfort of headache, fever, localized pain near the cheekbones or a sense of fullness, and the nasal discharge becomes thick and bad-smelling, sinus infection should be suspected. Nonprescription nosedrops and oral decongestants can be used for relief, but a prescription antibiotic is needed to eradicate the infection. Sometimes drainage of the sinuses is necessary if symptoms persist. Sinus infection can afflict children of all ages, with somewhat different presentations. For instance, a child under three years of age is likely to develop cellulitis around the eye, whereas an older child may have a paranasal or frontal sinusitis.

Medicines for Breathing Difficulties

Antihistamines

BROMPHENIRAMINE

Trade Name: Dimetane.

Dosage Forms: Sustained-release and regular tablet, elixir.

Available in Generic Form: Not as a single product.

Why Used: An antihistamine that dries up the mucous secretion in the nasal cavities as well as in the pharynx and the bronchial tree.

How to Give: Read and follow the dosage and instructions for use on the label.

Time to Take Effect: One to four hours.

Unintended Effects: Dry mouth and drowsiness are common.

Drug and Food Interactions: Medicines with sedative properties add to the drowsiness effect of this drug.

Contraindication: Use with caution in children with uncontrollable seizures or asthma.

Special Note: Useful for the relief of hay fever and allergy symptoms such as sneezing, itching and watery eyes.

Age Limitation: Not recommended for children under two years.

Storage Instruction: Keep at room temperature and the mouth of the bottle clean from syrup residues, otherwise the lid may get stuck to the bottle.

CHLORPHENIRAMINE

Trade Names: Aller-Chlor, Alermine, Chlorpheniramine, Chlo-Amine, Chlor-Niramine, Chlortrimeton, Teldrin.

Dosage Forms: Sustained-release chewable and regular tablet, sustained-release capsule, syrup, injection.

Available in Generic Form: Yes.

Why Used: An antihistamine that dries the mucous secretion in the nasal cavities as well as in the pharynx and the bronchial tree.

How to Give: Read and follow the dosage and instructions for use on the label.

Time to Take Effect: One to four hours.

Unintended Effects: Dry mouth and drowsiness are common.

Drug and Food Interactions: Medicines with sedative properties add to the drowsiness effect of this drug.

Contraindication: Use with caution in children with uncontrollable seizure or asthma.

Special Note: Useful for the relief of hay fever and allergy symptoms such as sneezing, itching and watery eyes.

Age Limitation: Not recommended for children under two years.

Storage Instruction: Keep at room temperature and the mouth of the bottle clean from syrup residues, otherwise the lid may get stuck to the bottle.

PYRILAMINE

Trade Names: Nervine, Nytol, Relax-U, Sominex. It is also a common ingredient in many combination cold remedies, such as Allerest, Cenagesic, Covanamine, Duadacin, Ginsopan, Valihist, Ventilade.

Dosage Forms: Tablet, sustained-release and regular capsule, liquid.

Available in Generic Form: Yes.

Why Used: An antihistamine that dries the mucous secretion in the nasal cavities as well as in the pharynx and the bronchial tree. Because it causes drowsiness, it is also used as a sleep aid.

How to Give: Read and follow the dosage and instructions for use on the label.

Time to Take Effect: One to two hours.

Unintended Effects:

- Dry mouth and drowsiness are common.
- Occasionally, nausea, vomiting, and loss of appetite.

Drug and Food Interaction: No significant interaction reported.

Contraindication: Use with caution in children with uncontrollable seizures or asthma.

Special Notes:

- The question of the possible cancer-causing effect of pyrilamine has been raised; however, there is no conclusive evidence to prove that it is not safe.
- Useful for the relief of allergy symptoms.

Age Limitation: Not recommended for children under two years.

Storage Instruction: Keep at room temperature.

Cough Medicines

CODEINE

Trade Names: Dispensed as a single product, codeine is a controlled drug that requires a prescription. However, it is a common ingredient in many combination cough medicines. Examples are: Baytussin AC, Cetro-Cirose, Calcidrine, Cotussis, Glydeine, Guiamid A.C., Halotussin w/Codeine, Liquitussin A.C., Nortussin w/Codeine, Robitussin A-C, SK-Terpin Hydrate and Codeine, Terpin Hydrate w/Codeine, Tolu-Sed.

Dosage Forms: Cough medicines are available in liquid form, whereas the prescription drug is available in tablet and injection forms.

Available in Generic Form: Yes.

Why Used: To decrease pain or cough.

How to Give:

- Take with food to alleviate discomfort to the stomach.
- Take only as needed rather than at regularly scheduled intervals, unless instructed otherwise by your health care provider.

Time to Take Effect: One to two hours.

Unintended Effects:

- Drowsiness, lightheadedness, and sedation are common.
- May cause upset stomach and constipation.
- Skin rash is a rare unintended effect.

Drug and Food Interactions:

- The drowsiness effect is increased by the use of other agents with sedative properties at the same time, e.g., cold remedies.
- Codeine intensifies the intoxicating effect of alcohol.

Contraindications: Previous allergy to this drug or other members of the opiate family, for example, meperidine and morphine.

Special Notes:

- This drug may be habit forming if used for prolonged periods (weeks to months).
- Tolerance to the sedative effect of this drug varies—the same dose may have different effects on different children.
- Encourage fluid intake with each dose to reduce the constipating effect.
- Consult your health care provider if your child's cough persists for more than three to four days.
- Some of the codeine-containing cough medicines also have a high content of alcohol, which may be undesirable for your child. Be sure to look for the alcohol content on the label of the bottle when selecting a cough medicine for your child.

Age Limitation: Not recommended for children under two years unless prescribed by a health care provider.

Storage Instruction: Keep at room temperature, in the case of a cough syrup; keep the mouth of the bottle clean from syrup residues, otherwise the lid may get stuck to the bottle.

DEXTROMETHORPHAN

Trade Names: Pertussin 8-Hour. It is a common ingredient in many combination cough remedies, such as Cheracol D, Codimal DM, Colrex, Consotuss, Coryban-D, Cosanyl DM Improved Formula, Formula 44-D, 2/G-DM, Novahistine DMX, Nyquil, Robitussin DM, Romilar Children's, St. Joseph's Cough Syrup for Children, Triaminicol, Vicks, Hold, Spec-T Sore Throat/Cough Suppressant, Vicks Formula-44 Cough Discs.

Dosage Forms: Liquid, lozenge.

Available in Generic Form: Yes.

Why Used: A nonnarcotic antitussive that inhibits coughing without pain-relief or addictive properties.

How to Give: Read and follow the dosage and instructions for use on the label.

Time to Take Effect: One to two hours.

Unintended Effect: None when used in recommended dose.

Contraindication: Previous allergy to this drug.

Drug and Food Interaction: No significant interaction reported.

Special Notes:

- The effective anticough dose is between 10 to 30 mg per dose and needs to be adjusted individually on the basis of age and weight (for children two to six years, the total daily dose should not exceed 30 mg, whereas for children aged six to twelve, the total daily dose should not exceed 60 mg).
- Consult your health care provider if your child's cough persists for more than three to four days.

Storage Instruction: Keep at room temperature, in the case of a cough syrup; keep the mouth of the bottle clean from syrup residues, otherwise the lid may get stuck to the bottle.

DIPHENHYDRAMINE

Trade Name: Benadryl.

Dosage Form: Syrup, cream.

Available in Generic Form: Yes.

Why Used: It has both antihistaminic and antitussive properties. Because of its drowsiness effect, it is also used as a sleep aid. Its antihistaminic property dries the mucous secretion in the nasal cavities as well as in the pharynx and the bronchial tree and also suppresses coughing.

How to Give:

- Read and follow the dosage and instructions for use on the label.
- This medicine can be given with food.

Time to Take Effect: One to two hours.

Unintended Effect: Dry mouth and drowsiness are common.

Drug and Food Interaction: No significant interaction reported.

Contraindications:

- Use with caution in children with uncontrollable seizures or asthma.
- Previous allergy to this drug (hypersensitivity can develop following the use of the topical cream).

Special Notes:

- Diphenhydramine is approved by the Food and Drug Administration as a nonprescription cough medicine and allergy remedy. It is also available in several brands of nonprescription sleep aids (Compoz, Nytol, Sominex Formula 2).
- The cream form of diphenhydramine has a high incidence of sensitizing effect—it can result in skin reactions such as hives, rash, and itchiness. For this reason avoid using this drug externally to treat an allergy condition such as reaction to poison oak.

Age Limitation: Not recommended for children under two years unless prescribed by a health care provider.

Storage Instruction: Keep at room temperature, in case of the syrup; keep the mouth of the bottle clean from syrup residues, otherwise the lid may get stuck to the bottle.

GUAIFENESIN

Trade Names: Anti-Tuss, Baytussin, Breonesin, Colrex, Gee-Gee, GG-Cen, GG-Tussin, Glycotuss, Glytuss, G-200, Hytuss, Hytuss-2X, Liquitussin, Malotuss, Nortussin, Robitussin, S-T Expectorant, 2/G.

Dosage Forms: Tablet, capsule, syrup.

Available in Generic Form: Yes.

Why Used: An expectorant that promotes or facilitates the evacuation of secretions from the bronchial airways to provide temporary relief of coughs due to minor throat and bronchial irritation as may occur with upper respiratory infection, it also reduces the thickness of these secretions by increasing the formation of a more fluid secretion.

How to Give: Read and follow the dosage and instructions for use on the label.

Time to Take Effect: One to two hours.

Unintended Effect: Rarely may cause stomach discomfort.

Contraindication: Previous allergy to this drug.

Drug and Food Interaction: No significant interaction reported.

Special Notes:

- Fluid intake enhances the expectorant effect of this drug. Encourage your child to drink as much fluid as possible while taking this drug.
- Consult your health care provider if your child's cough persists for more than three to four days.
- Some expectorants may contain alcohol in the syrup. If that is not desirable for your child, be sure to look for the alcohol content on the label of the bottle when selecting an expectorant.

Age Limitation: Not recommended for children under two years.

Storage Instruction: Keep at room temperature, and keep the mouth of the bottle clean from syrup residue; otherwise, the lid may get stuck to the bottle.

Decongestants

OXYMETAZOLINE

Trade Names: Afrin, Bayfrin, Dristan Long Lasting, Duramist Plus, Duration, Neosynephrine 12 Hour, Nostrilla, Oxymetazoline, Sinex Long-Lasting.

Dosage Forms: Nasal drug and spray.

Available in Generic Form: Yes.

Why Used: A long-acting decongestant that reduces nasal congestion by constricting dilated blood vessels within the nasal cavities, thus temporarily reducing the swelling associated with inflammation of the mucous membrane lining the nasal passage.

How to Give: Read and follow the dosage and instructions for use on the label. For a more detailed discussion on how to give medicines by nose, see Chapter 4.

Time to Take Effect: Thirty minutes to one hour.

Unintended Effects: Rarely, nervousness, dizziness, and insomnia may occur.

Drug and Food Interaction: No significant interaction reported.

Contraindications:

- Use with caution in diabetics or in the presence of high blood pressure.
- Previous allergy to this drug.

Special Notes:

- An effective topical decongestant that may last eight to twelve hours after each application.
- Do not use for more than five days consecutively, to avoid increasing the likelihood of *rebound congestion* (see Glossary). If this medicine is needed beyond five days, stop and rest for two days before using it again.
- It is a common ingredient in many combination decongestants for oral use.

Age Limitation: Not recommended for children under two years. Only drops should be used in children two to six years old, since the spray is difficult to use in the small nostril.

Storage Instruction: Keep at room temperature.

PHENYLEPHRINE

Trade Names: Alconefrin 12, Alconefrin 25, Alconefrin 50, Allerest Nasal, Coricidin Nasal Mist, Duration Mild, Neo-Synephrine, Nostril, Sinarest Nasal, Sinex, Vacon.

Dosage Forms: Nasal drop and spray.

Available in Generic Form: Yes.

Why Used: A decongestant that reduces nasal congestion by constricting dilated blood vessels within the nasal cavities, it temporarily reduces the swelling associated with inflammation of the mucous membrane lining the nasal passage.

How to Give: Read and follow the dosage and instructions for use on the label. For a detailed discussion on how to give medicines by nose, see Chapter 4.

Time to Take Effect: Thirty minutes to one hour.

Unintended Effect: The incidence of *rebound congestion* (see Glossary) is more common with this drug than when using the long-acting topical decongestant.

Drug and Food Interaction: No significant interaction reported.

Contraindications:

- Previous allergy to this drug.
- Use with caution in children with severe heart disease.

Special Notes:

- An effective topical decongestant except for its relatively short duration of action.
- Do not use for more than five days consecutively, to avoid increasing the likelihood of *rebound congestion* (see Glossary). If this medicine is needed beyond five days, stop and rest for two days before using it again.

Age Limitation: May be used in children under two years.

Storage Instruction: Keep at room temperature.

PHENYLPROPANOLAMINE

Trade Names: Decongestant-P, Phenylpropanolamine, Propadrine, Propagest, Rhindecon. It is also a common ingredient in many combination oral decongestant products, such as Allerest, Bayer Children's Cold Tablets, Bayer Decongestant, Contac, Coricidin D, Coryban-D, Novahistine, Ornex, Sine-Off, Sinurex, Sinustate, Sinutab, St. Joseph's Cold Tablets for Children, Super Anahist, Triaminic, Triaminicin.

Dosage Forms: Sustained-release and regular capsule, tablet, syrup, elixir.

Available in Generic Form: Yes.

Why Used: A decongestant that reduces nasal congestion by constricting dilated blood vessels within the nasal cavities, it temporarily reduces the swelling associated with inflammation of the mucous membrane lining the nasal passage.

How to Give: Read and follow the dosage and instructions for use on the label. For a detailed discussion on how to give medicines by nose, see Chapter 4.

Time to Take Effect: Thirty minutes to one hour.

Drug and Food Interaction: No significant interaction reported.

Unintended Effects: Occasionally, restlessness and insomnia.

Contraindications:

- Previous allergy to this drug.

- Use with caution in the presence of severe heart disease and high blood pressure.

Special Notes:

- This drug is used in some nonprescription diet aids because of its stimulant effect on the brain. It is also a common ingredient in some illicit street drugs known as speed.
- When used judiciously and instructions are followed properly, its stimulant effect is hardly noticeable.

Age Limitation: Not recommended for children under two years.

Storage Instruction: Keep at room temperature.

PSEUDOEPHEDRINE

Trade Names: Cenafed, Kodet SE, Neo-Fed, Neo-Synephrinol Day, Novafed, Pseudoephedrine, Sudafed, Sudrin.

Dosage Forms: Tablet, sustained-release tablet, liquid.

Available in Generic Form: Yes.

Why Used: A decongestant that reduces nasal congestion by constricting dilated blood vessels within the nasal cavities, it temporarily reduces the swelling associated with inflammation of the mucous membrane lining the nasal passage.

How to Give: Read and follow the dosage and instructions for use on the label.

Time to Take Effect: Thirty minutes to one hour.

Unintended Effects: Rarely, headache and insomnia may occur.

Contraindications:

- Previous allergy to this drug.
- Use with caution in the presence of severe heart disease and high blood pressure.

Drug and Food Interaction: No significant interaction reported.

Special Notes: When this drug is used judiciously and the instructions are followed properly, its unintended effects are hardly noticeable.

Age Limitation: Not recommended for children under two years.

Storage Instruction: Keep at room temperature.

CHAPTER 10

Medicines for the Eye

Anatomy of the Eye

The human eye is a remarkable and delicate organ. It is situated in a bony cavity called the orbit. The bony front portion of the orbit is strong, whereas the bony side wall is very thin. The internal orbit has openings that allow the optic nerve to pass directly into the brain.

Eye movements are controlled by the extraocular muscles and coordinated by the brain. These muscles are responsible for the movement of both eyes so that they move together no matter where the child looks.

The eye itself is a sphere that holds a fluid-filled center. The fluid gives the eye its shape, and the external supporting tissue layers give it strength. If this surrounding supporting tissue is injured or cut, the fluid escapes and the eye collapses, much like air being let out of a balloon.

As you look at the human eye, you can see the following structures: the brow, which is composed of skin and hair over the edge of the orbit; the upper and lower eyelids, which are made up of some of the thinnest skin in your child's body. Muscles, ligaments, connective tissue, and fat hold and support the eye within the orbit. The eyelids also serve as a protective covering for the eyes. The lid margins are lined with hairs and oil-secreting glands. The hairs help protect the eye. The inner part of the eyelids is lined with a thin mucous membrane called the conjunctiva. It is pink and shiny.

The cornea is a thin, completely clear tissue that lines the front or external portion of the eye. It focuses and transmits light to the interior

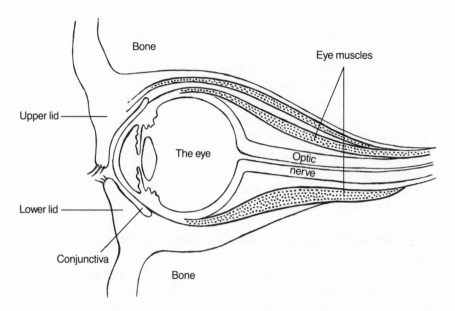

This cross section shows the eye in the bony cavity and how it is supported by the muscles and connective tissue.

of the eye. It is composed of cells that protect the eye. The sclera or white part you see as you look at your child's eye is continuous with the cornea and encircles the eye completely.

The iris is the colored portion of the eye. The color of your child's eyes is determined by genes from both the father and the mother. The hole in the center of the iris is called the pupil. The iris controls the amount of light entering the eye by dilating or opening in dim light and contracting or closing in bright light.

The eye itself is divided into two segments: the front or anterior

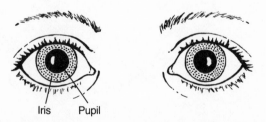

The pupil is the dark center of the human eye. The iris is the colored area.

segment and the rear or posterior segment. There is a clear fluid in both segments. The lens is in the posterior segment, right behind the iris. It focuses light onto the retina. Lining the posterior of the eye is the retina. It consists of a complex and specialized network of nerve fibers and cells that transmit light and images to the optic nerve. The optic nerve then transmits the message to the brain. The retina recognizes dim light through visual cells called rods. Color is identified by cells in the retina called cones. When visual impulses enter the optic nerve, they travel over a pathway to an area of the brain designed to receive and interpret the images.

Tears protect your child's eyes. They lubricate, hydrate, and remove foreign substances from the eye. Tearing also protects the eye from infection. Tears are produced by the lacrimal glands, the largest of which lies in the upper temporal area of the eye orbit. Another gland lies alongside the nose on the inner aspect of the eye. These glands are not visible unless they are swollen. The larger lacrimal sac has a duct inside the eyelids that permits an overflow of tears to enter the nose, which explains why your nose runs when you cry.

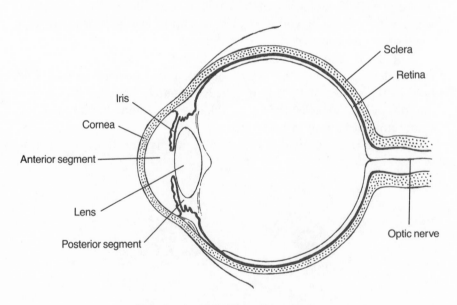

The structures that form the eyeball.

It is important to seek medical attention if you notice any abnormalities in or around the eyes. This is not simply because sight is so important but because the eye is also one organ that leads directly to the brain, so that injury or infection may harm brain tissue in addition to the eye.

Development of the Eye

When a baby is born, the iris color is slate blue in light-skinned infants and deep brown in children of dark skin. The final color of the iris is established during the first three to six months of life. The pupil of the infant's eye is small and slow to dilate; this is why newborns close their eyes in direct bright light such as sunshine or a camera flash. The pupil becomes more reactive as the infant grows older.

At birth the child's eye is about three-quarters the size of an adult's eye. It grows rapidly during the first year of life and continues to grow at a slower pace until puberty, when it reaches adult proportions. The ability to fixate both eyes at the same time is not well developed at birth. However, this improves, and proper eye fixation should be achieved by three to four months of age. If your child has one eye that deviates markedly from the object being observed, this may indicate that your child is cross-eyed. This condition needs to be evaluated by a

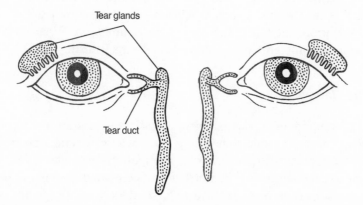

The lacrimal glands, which produce **tears**, lie along the outer, upper edge of the eye and along the nose.

physician or ophthalmologist (doctor who specializes in eye problems), because it can indicate a serious eye problem or disorder.

At birth the infant cannot clearly visualize objects like adults can, since vision is about 20/600. However, the child can discriminate large objects such as the human face. By about two to two and a half months of age, an infant's eyes should be able to follow a brightly colored object for 180 degrees. Recent research by Dr. T. Berry Brazelton has shown that newborns as young as a few days old, when held within eight to twelve inches from an adult's face, can mimic facial expressions made by the adult.

The newborn infant sheds no tears when crying. Tears are usually not formed in enough quantity to overflow the eyelids until about the second or third month of life. If your infant is tearing excessively when not crying, it may indicate an obstruction of the tear duct and needs an evaluation by a physician.

When your child is examined by a nurse practitioner or physician in infancy and early childhood, the eyes are checked with an instrument called an ophthalmoscope. The National Society for the Prevention of Blindness recommends that by three to four years of age the child should have a first eye exam by an ophthalmologist.

Common Eye Problems

Some of the most common types of eye injuries and diseases that are seen in children from infancy to adolescence are presented in this section. Since the eye is such a delicate structure, do not self-medicate most eye problems but rather seek medical attention. What may seem like a minor problem could lead to visual impairment.

In the Newborn

The trauma of a vaginal birth occasionally results in edema, or swelling, of the eyelids, but this goes down in several days without treatment. Some infants also display red spots on the white sclera, which are called subconjunctival hemorrhages. These are due to the trauma of birth causing rupture of small capillaries (blood vessels) in the sclera. This is normal and does not harm the eyes; the spots disappear in several weeks. Some infants react to eye medicine that is instilled in all infants' eyes shortly after birth to prevent infection. It may cause reddening of the conjunctiva. This also should clear on its own in several days.

If your infant is shedding excessive tears when not crying, this needs to be evaluated by a physician. Some infants experience blocked tear ducts, which require medical attention. This is demonstrated by excess tearing because the tears are produced but do not pass through the blocked duct to drain out of the eye.

Foreign Bodies and Injuries

One of the best ways to handle eye injuries is to prevent them. This means inspecting toys for sharp or hazardous parts, supervising toy usage, and keeping caustic agents out of your child's reach. Teach your child to properly use and respect sports and household equipment and to use tools properly. This helps the child learn how to protect the eyes and sight. Injuries are the leading cause of blindness in children over two years of age.

Foreign bodies in the eye of an infant or small child are usually noted by irritability, tearing, and rubbing of the eye. The older child is able to tell you of the problem by complaining of pain or burning. In order to visualize the eye adequately, you need to have the child lie down, restraining the younger child as necessary. Gently grasp the eyelashes with your fingers and open the lids by pulling the upper lid upward and the lower lid downward. Inspect the eye carefully. A child who is old enough to follow instructions can assist by focusing the eyes up, down, far left, and far right. When you locate the piece of foreign material, assess whether you can safely remove it without damaging your child's eye. Does the object appear to be freely moveable? Never try to remove anything that has penetrated the eye itself.

If the foreign object can be removed, use a piece of sterile gauze that you have folded and moistened with saline solution. Gently touch it to the object, and remove it from the eye. If the object cannot be removed by touching it, do not apply pressure to the gauze and try to move it out of the eye, because you could scratch the delicate tissue.

Sterile gauze can be purchased at the drugstore. It is individually packaged so that each piece has no germs. If you carefully remove it from its wrapping so as not to touch the corner that you will place in the eye, you will not introduce germs into the eye. Saline solution can also be purchased at the drugstore. Buy the type that is used as wetting solution for hard contact lenses or storage solution for soft contact lenses, because it is similar to the tear solution in the eye. If you do not have these things on hand, you can use a clean tissue that has been moistened with running tap water.

Another method is to use a sterile saline solution to irrigate the eye. This may work more effectively with a young child or infant. Remember not to put the solution directly on the cornea but, rather, place it on the inner corner closest to the nose and flush toward the outer corner of the eye. This is achieved by directing the flow of fluid from the bottle toward the outer edge of the eye.

If the object appears to be sharp, such as wood chips or sand, it could have scratched the cornea. In this case the child's eyes should be checked for possible abrasions by a physician.

Penetrating injuries usually occur from trauma caused by stones, sharp toys, arrows, air rifles, or any sharp or blunt object entering the eye. It is important to remember never to remove an object that has penetrated the eye. Observe the child for fluid leaking out of the eye. Lie the child down with the head elevated about thirty degrees. Cover the eye with a sterile gauze pad or clean towel, and cover the uninjured eye also to reduce eye movement, since both eyes move together. Remain calm, comfort the child, and get to the nearest medical facility immediately. Do not put any ointment or drops into the eye. Do prevent the child from rubbing the eye.

Chemical Injuries

Chemical injuries most commonly occur when a toddler dumps something into the eye or something explodes in the face of an older child. You need to act quickly, because chemical damage continues to occur until the chemicals are flushed from the eye. Have the child lie down, restraining him or her as necessary. Gently grasp the eyelashes or lids with your fingers and open the lids by gently pulling the upper lid upward and lower lid downward. Immediately irrigate the eye with a prepackaged saline solution or tap water for fifteen minutes, by simply pouring water from a container such as a cup over the eye continuously for the entire fifteen minutes. Again, it is best not to put the solution directly on the cornea but, rather, place it on the inner corner closest to the nose and flush toward the outer corner of the eye. Do not put any ointment or drops into the eye, but do get your child to a medical facility immediately following the irrigation. If possible, bring the container or agent that caused the injury to the medical facility with you. A delay of seconds can increase the extent of the chemical damage to the delicate eye tissue.

Sun Injuries

Sunburn can cause irritation to the cornea, with actual loss of corneal cells. If the child is in pain after exposure to bright sunlight, consult your health care provider.

Infections of the Eye

Children are susceptible to eye infections. Some of the most common types are discussed here. All the possible infections are not discussed here, and if you notice that your child has complaints of eye pain or discomfort that are not described here, do not hesitate to see your health care provider as soon as possible.

Conjunctivitis

Conjunctivitis, or pinkeye, is one of the most common childhood eye infections. It may or may not be infectious to others with whom the child has contact. The eyelids may be swollen, with a thick, puslike discharge from the eye, which may cause the eye to be matted shut when the child awakens. The conjunctiva appears red, and your child usually feels like his or her eyes are burning or has something in them. This should be treated by a health care provider. Usually an antibiotic eye ointment is prescribed. See Chapter 4 for a description of how to instill eye medicines.

Epidemic Keratoconjunctivitis

This form of conjunctivitis is caused by a virus and is highly contagious. It usually occurs with children under two. It is spread by coughing or direct contact. The eye is very red or pink and has a sensation of itching and burning. It becomes sensitive to light, a condition called photophobia. In 50 percent of the cases there are also flulike symptoms. Prevent your child from rubbing the eyes and contact your health care provider for treatment.

Allergic Conjunctivitis

Allergic conjunctivitis is usually seasonal and is characterized by itching, tearing, and some swelling of the lids. Its cause, as the name implies, is allergy. Some relief from symptoms can be obtained by applying cool compresses to the eyes. You can do this by placing a clean washcloth moistened with cool tap water over the child's closed eyelids for five to ten minutes. If your child is rubbing the eyes, unable to get relief from the cool compresses, or if the symptoms worsen, consult your health care provider.

Chemical Conjunctivitis

This is caused by contact with irritating chemicals such as sprays, fumes, smoke, or pollutants in the air. The eyes need to be irrigated immediately with normal saline or tap water for fifteen minutes. See the section on chemical eye injuries earlier in this chapter for the procedure to be followed for eye irrigation. If discomfort persists after irrigation or if you have questions about whether the cornea was damaged, contact your health care provider.

Blepharitis

Blepharitis is an inflammation of the eyelid margins, characterized by redness, scaling, burning, or itching. There are two common types. *Bacterial* blepharitis is usually caused by the staphylococcus organism. The scales are hard and tenacious, so they are difficult to remove. *Seborrheic* blepharitis is seen in combination with dermatitis of the scalp, brow, or external ears. With this type the scales are greasy and easy to remove. Both eyelids are usually involved. It is important to consult your health care provider so the type of blepharitis can be diagnosed and properly treated.

Hordeolum or Stye

A stye is a painful swelling and infection of the lid at the lash line. This should be seen by a health care provider to assess the need for treatment. A stye usually gets better in several days if treated with warm compresses. Usually the compresses are prescribed to be used three to four times a day for fifteen to twenty minutes at a time. An antibiotic ointment may also be prescribed. If untreated, the stye could lead to a generalized infection of the eyelid. Never squeeze the eyelid because this sends the infectious material into the lid tissue.

Chalazion or Internal Stye

A chalazion is a painless swelling of a gland in the eyelid (meibomian). The eyelid has a visible raised bump on the lid that varies in size according to the amount of swelling of the gland involved. This tends to occur more often on the inner aspects of the eyelid than the hordeolum (stye), with the swelling being cystlike and generally not painful. The symptoms tend to recur and need to be evaluated by a health care provider.

Contact Lenses

Some older children choose to use contact lenses for cosmetic reasons or because they often improve the visual acuity more than glasses.

Understanding the care and maintenance of these lenses is necessary to prevent eye injury. This is true for both hard and soft lenses. Proper cleaning and storage of the lenses minimizes the chance of eye infections. Care must include using a proper lens solution. Some children may experience a sensitivity to a preservative found in a lens solution. By careful reading of the label, your child can avoid the offending lens solution in the future. Meticulous care of the contact lens case should be taken, and the solution in the case must be changed daily.

Injury can be done to the cornea if the lenses are not properly cared for. One of the common problems is wearing the lenses too long or sleeping with lenses not designed for that purpose. This causes corneal swelling because the contact lens blocks the oxygen supply to the cornea. The corneal tissue cannot repair itself without adequate oxygen. Red and watering eyes are a sign of eye irritation in the contact wearer.

Eye Reactions to Makeup

Young girls may experience allergic reactions to makeup, causing the lids to become reddened and irritated. All makeup needs to be fully removed each day before going to bed. This reduces eye irritation. Hypoallergenic eye makeup may also reduce allergic reactions.

Makeup can become contaminated by germs because of improper handling, length of time used (over six months), and the chemical formulation of the cosmetic. Discard all makeup that is contaminated or is over a year old. Using eye makeup belonging to someone else can cause or spread eye infections. If your daughter has an eye infection, she should be advised against wearing eye makeup until the problem is resolved.

Eye Medicines

Self-medication with nonprescription eye drugs should only be undertaken for very minor eye problems. Most nonprescription eye medicines only relieve symptoms rather than curing the underlying cause. Since most parents do not have the expertise to diagnose eye problems or the equipment necessary to visualize the internal eye structures, it is difficult to find the cause of an eye problem. Any eye problem that does not respond to home treatment in forty-eight hours needs to be evaluated by a health care provider. Also any acutely painful eye problem or change in visual acuity needs immediate evaluation either by a physician or an ophthalmologist.

The Food and Drug Administration (FDA) recommends that only the following minor eye problems be treated with nonprescription medicines: dry eye, corneal edema in children, minor inflammation and irritation, and foreign bodies in the eye.

Dry Eye

Chronic dry eye is a condition seen mostly in older people; it rarely occurs in children. Wind, sun, chemical irritants, or illness can decrease the amount of tears in the eye, which needs to be bathed in tears to protect the delicate tissue. When there is a decreased or insufficient tear secretion, the eye feels dry and irritated and may appear red. If this is a chronic problem, your child needs to be evaluated by a health care provider.

Medicines for Dry Eye

Table 5   Cellulose Wetting Agents

Main Ingredient	Trade Names
Hydroxyethylcellulose	Absorbotear, Lyteers
Hydroxypropyl methylcellulose	Isopto Alkaline, Isopto Plain, Lacril, Muro Tears, Tearisol, Ultra Tears
Methylcellulose	Methopto ¼%, Methopto-Forte ½%, Methopto-Forte 1%, Milroy Artificial Tears, Murine Eye Drops, Murocel Ophthalmic Solution, Visculose-1%

Dosage Form: Eyedrops.

Why Used: To hold water and slow the movement of tears across the eye. These products are the most viscous cellulose derivative solutions, which are retained in the eye twice as long as saline solutions.

How to Give: Administer eyedrops as directed in Chapter 4. Instill the number of drops as directed by the manufacturer. Do not touch the dispenser tip to lashes, eye, or hands due to possibility of contamination. Remove contact lenses prior to use.

Unintended Effects:

- Dry crusts tend to form on eyelids, but these are harmless and can be wiped away with sterile gauze.
- May build up film on contact lenses.

Contraindications:

- Previous allergy to these ingredients or preservatives or any other agents in this product.
- Do not use this product with a prescription eye medicine without first contacting your health care provider.

Drug and Food Interactions: Check with health care prescriber before use with prescription eye preparations.

Special Notes:

- If the eye condition continues for forty-eight hours with use, discontinue and seek the advice of a health care provider at once.

- Do not use any solutions that are cloudy or discolored. Discard any solution within three months from the date of opening. Most medications are outdated after this time or become contaminated. If an opened bottle of eye solution has crystals on the lip or tip of the dispenser, do not use because of the danger of introducing crystals into the eye.

Age Limitations: Consult health care provider for use in children under two years.

Storage Instruction: Store at room temperature in a locked, secure medicine container out of reach of children.

POLYVINYL ALCOHOL

Trade Names: Liquifilm Forte, Liquifilm Tears, Tears Plus.

Dosage Forms: Eyedrops.

Why Used: It forms a protective film to soothe the eye by keeping it moist and lubricated. Less viscous than cellulose-containing medicines. Used in hard contact lens solutions to decrease eye irritation.

How to Give: Administer eyedrops as directed in Chapter 4. Instill the number of drops as directed by the manufacturer. Do not touch the dispenser tip to lashes, eye, or hands due to possibility of contamination. Remove contact lenses prior to use.

Unintended Effects: A sensitivity reaction of local redness and irritation is rare.

Contraindications:

- Do not use eye products containing alkaline borate with polyvinyl alcohol eye products because it can form gummy deposits in the eye.
- Previous allergy to this ingredient or preservatives or any other agent in this product.
- Do not use this product with a prescription eye medicine without first contacting your health care provider.

Drug and Food Interactions: Check with health care prescriber before use with prescription eye preparations.

Special Notes:

- If the eye condition continues for forty-eight hours with use, discontinue and seek the advise of a health care provider at once.

- Do not use any solutions that are cloudy or discolored. Discard any solution within three months from the date of opening. Most medications are outdated after this time or become contaminated. If an opened bottle of eye solution has crystals on the lip or tip of the dispenser, do not use because of the danger of introducing crystals into the eye.

Age Limitations: Consult health care provider for use in children under two years.

Storage Instruction: Store at room temperature in a locked, secure medicine container out of reach of children.

Corneal Edema

Edema is the medical term for swelling. When the cornea absorbs too much fluid, swelling results. It is usually indicative of an underlying eye problem that requires a physician's evaluation and treatment. If your child complains of blurred vision, seeing halos around lights, sensitivity to light, or pain, corneal edema may be the cause and your child should be seen by a health care provider immediately.

Inflammation and Irritation of the Eye

When substances such as dust, pollen, pollutants, chlorinated swimming pool water, or any foreign substances get into the eye, they cause blinking, tearing, redness, and discomfort. Allergies often produce the same symptoms. Medicines that are decongestants and vasoconstrictors, which constrict the blood vessels of the white portion of the eye, reducing redness, are to be used only on a short-term basis for minor eye problems and should not be used regularly. Continued treatment may mask the symptoms of a potential eye disease in your child. If the condition does not improve in forty-eight hours, consult your health care provider.

Decongestants and Vasoconstrictors

NAPHAZOLINE HYDROCHLORIDE IN CONCENTRATIONS OF 0.01% TO 0.03%

Trade Names: Allerest Eye Drops, Clear Eyes, Degest 2, Naphcon, Vaso-Clear.

Dosage Forms: Eyedrops.

Why Used: A vasoconstrictor, which constricts the blood vessels of the sclera (the white portion of the eye), it reduces redness.

How to Give: Administer eyedrops as directed in Chapter 4. Instill the number of drops as directed by the manufacturer. Do not touch the dispenser tip to lashes, eye, or hands due to possibility of contamination. Remove contact lenses prior to use.

Unintended Effects:

- If overused or used in higher concentrations than recommended by the manufacturer, it can dilate the pupil, making the eye sensitive to light.
- It may also cause the blood vessels to dilate, making the eye appear red. This is known as the rebound effect; the medicine must be stopped or the eye will remain red and irritated.

Contraindications:

- Do not use if child has glaucoma or other serious eye disease.
- Previous allergy to this ingredient or preservatives or any other agent in this product.

Drug and Food Interactions: Do not use this product with prescription eye preparations without first contacting health care provider.

Special Notes:

- Seek medical care if condition persists over forty-eight hours.
- Do not use any solutions that are cloudy or discolored. Discard any solution within three months from the date of opening. Most medications are outdated after this time or become contaminated. If an opened bottle of eye solution has crystals on the lip or tip of the dispenser, do not use because of the danger of introducing crystals into the eye.

Age Limitations: Consult health care provider for use in children under six years.

Storage Instruction: Store at room temperature in a locked, secure medicine container out of reach of children. If taken internally, can cause central nervous system excitement (nervousness and irritability).

PHENYLEPHRINE HYDROCHLORIDE IN CONCENTRATIONS
OF 0.08% TO 0.2%

Trade Names: Eye Cool, Isopto-Frin, Optigene II Eye Drops, Phenylzin, Prefrin Liquifilm, Soothe, Tear-efrin Eye Drops, Zincfrin.

Dosage Forms: Eyedrops.

Why Used: Constricts blood vessels of the sclera (the white portion of the eye) to reduce redness.

How to Give: Administer eyedrops as directed in Chapter 4. Instill the number of drops as directed by the manufacturer. Do not touch the dispenser tip to lashes, eye, or hands due to possibility of contamination. Remove contact lenses prior to use.

Unintended Effects:

- If overused or used in higher concentrations than recommended by the manufacturer, it can dilate the pupil, making the eye sensitive to light.
- It may also cause the blood vessels to dilate, making the eye appear red. This is known as the rebound effect. The medicine must be stopped or the eye will remain red and irritated.

Contraindications:

- Do not use if your child has glaucoma or other serious eye diseases.
- Previous allergy to this ingredient or preservatives or any other agent in this product.
- Do not use with soft contact lenses.

Drug and Food Interactions: Do not use this product with a prescription eye medicine without first contacting your health care provider.

Special Notes:

- If redness persists over forty-eight hours, consult a physician at once.
- The effectiveness is variable, because the drug is unstable after being opened due to chemical changes occurring when the drug contacts air. Keep the lid on tight and do not transfer the eyedrops to any container other than the original bottle.
- Do not use any solutions that are cloudy or discolored. Discard any solution within three months from the date of opening. Most medications are outdated after this time or become contaminated. If an opened bottle of eye solution has crystals on the lip or tip of the dispenser do not use because of the danger of introducing crystals into the eye.

Age Limitations: Consult health care provider for use in children under six years.

Storage Instruction: Store at room temperature in a locked, secure medicine container out of reach of children. If taken internally it can cause central nervous system excitement (nervousness and irritability).

Tetrahydrozoline Hydrochloride in Concentrations of 0.05%

Trade Names: Clear & Brite, Murine Plus Eye Drops, Optigene III, Soothe Eye Drops, Tetrasine, Visine, Visine A.C.

Dosage Forms: Eyedrops.

Why Used: Constricts blood vessels of the sclera (the white portion of the eye) to reduce redness.

How to Give: Administer eyedrops as directed in Chapter 4. Instill the number of drops as directed by the manufacturer. Do not touch the dispenser tip to lashes, eye, or hands due to possibility of contamination. Remove contact lenses prior ω use.

Unintended Effects: Rare, because it does not dilate the pupils. No report of rebound congestion with use in the eye.

Contraindications:

- Do not use if your child has glaucoma or other serious eye diseases.
- Previous allergy to this ingredient or preservatives or any other agent in this product.

Drug and Food Interactions: Do not use this product with a prescription eye medicine without first contacting your health care provider.

Special Notes:

- Seek medical care if redness persists over forty-eight hours.
- Do not use any solutions that are cloudy or discolored. Discard any solution within three months from the date of opening. Most medications are outdated after this time or become contaminated. If an opened bottle of eye solution has crystals on the lip or tip of the dispenser do not use because of the danger of introducing crystals into the eye.

Age Limitations: Consult health care provider for use in children under six years.

Storage Instruction: Store at room temperature in a locked, secure medicine container out of reach of children. If taken internally it can cause central nervous system excitement (nervousness and irritability).

Foreign Bodies in the Eye

EYE IRRIGANTS

Trade Names: A/K/Rinse, Blinx, Eye-Stream, Decriose, Lauro, Lavoptik Eye Wash, M/Rinse, Trisol Eye Wash.

Dosage Form: Eyewash.

Why Used: For eye irrigation.

How to Give: Administer eye irrigation as directed in Chapter 4. Contact health care provider or poison control following irrigation. Do not touch the dispenser tip to lashes, eye, or hands due to possibility of contamination. Remove contact lenses prior to use.

Unintended Effect: None.

Contraindication: Do not use if the eye has a penetrating injury.

Drug and Food Interactions: None.

Special Notes:

- This medicine duplicates normal tears and contains no active medicine.
- If severe eye pain continues, or if substance is not removed by flushing, or changes in vision occur such as floating spots, double vision, sensitivity to light, or if redness continues, consult your physician at once.
- Do not use any solutions that are cloudy or discolored. Discard any solution within three months from the date of opening. Most medications are outdated after this time or become contaminated. If an opened bottle of eye solution has crystals on the lip or tip of the dispenser, do not use because of the danger of introducing crystals into the eye.

Age Limitations: None.

Storage Instruction: Store at room temperature.

Other Eye Problems

Although the FDA states that hordeolum, commonly known as stye, blepharitis, and conjunctivitis may benefit from home treatment, these conditions in children should be treated by a physician. Since the child's eye is delicate, it is important to have prompt, accurate diagnosis and treatment to prevent any problems that could result in permanent eye damage. There is no nonprescription medicine for treatment of these conditions.

CHAPTER 11

Medicines for the Ear

Did you know that your newborn infant has been listening to your heartbeat and other uterine sounds for at least four months before birth? Studies have demonstrated that in addition to hearing, infants show a range of discriminative listening in response to certain sounds.

Aristotle wrote centuries ago that the ear is the organ of education. Rightly so, because through feedback from sound, learning is confirmed to the individual. Since a child's learning starts in early infancy, it is important that hearing be evaluated and protected.

Anatomy of the Ear

The External Ear

The part of the ear that you see on either side of your child's head is known as the external ear. The stiff, formed part of the external ear is made up of cartilage and skin and is called the auricle or pinna. The soft lobe at the bottom of the ear has no cartilage and is the only part of the ear to contain fatty tissue. The outer ear has a very rich blood supply.

Near the center of the ear is an opening called the external auditory canal. It is a long, tunnel-shaped area along which sound is transmitted to the eardrum or tympanic membrane. The ear canal is lined with sweat glands and tiny hairs. The sweat glands produce the waxy substance you know as ear wax. Ear wax functions to protect the delicate skin lining the canal and trap foreign particles. This wax is usually brown in color and quite soft. In most cases there is no need to remove this wax, because the hairs in the canal propel it to the end of the external ear canal, where it can safely be removed with a washcloth. Cotton-tipped applicators are not recommended to remove wax from your child's ears, since they tend to push the wax toward the eardrum, where it may form a hardened plug. Sharp objects such as bobby pins should never be used, because they can scratch the lining and expose the tissue to infection or even harm the eardrum.

The Middle Ear

The drumlike area known as the tympanic membrane is made up of several layers of tissue. It protects the fragile middle ear components and also magnifies sound. Inside the middle ear area is an air-filled chamber with a long tube leading from it called the eustachian or auditory tube. This tube equalizes pressure in this chamber. The eustachian tube leads into the back of the throat and is generally closed. However, if you swallow or yawn, the tube opens to maintain equal air pressure. You may remember that when you go to the mountains or fly in an airplane your ears feel full and sound seems distorted. To relieve this sensation you may hold your nose and blow, causing your ears to

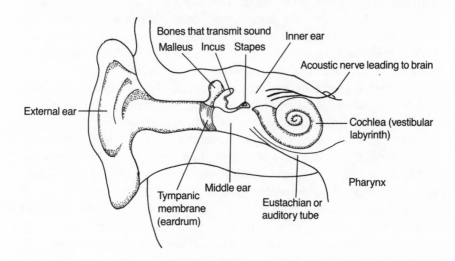

The anatomy of the ear.

pop, or you can yawn, swallow, or chew gum. All these methods open the eustachian tube and equalize pressure. An infant can equalize the pressure inside the ears by sucking on a bottle or pacifier as altitude is lost or gained.

The eustachian tube connects the middle ear to the throat. Because of this opening, infections can sometimes ascend from the mouth into the middle ear. This is especially true in the infant and young child, whose eustachian tubes are more horizontal. In the child over four, the eustachian tube has a slight angle that helps prevent infection.

The Inner Ear

Sound is transmitted to the inner ear by three of the smallest bones in the human body. They lie right behind the eardrum. You probably know them as the hammer, anvil, and stirrup. They are technically named the malleus, incus, and stapes.

The components of the inner ear are bathed in fluid. There is a large seashell-like device called the cochlea. Sound enters the middle ear through the oval windows, a small windowlike opening covered by the stapes, setting the fluid in the cochlea vibrating. Lining the cochlea are thousands of tiny hairs that are moved when sound strikes them. Through their movements, these hairs send messages to the acoustic nerve, which leads to the area of the brain designed to receive and identify sound messages. The hairs are fragile and can be damaged by trauma, infection, or drugs. If these hairs are damaged, hearing will be completely lost and not even a hearing aid can restore hearing.

Another component of the inner ear is the vestibular labyrinth, which maintains the sense of balance and equilibrium. The inner ear plays an important part in balance as well as hearing.

Hearing is not a simple process. Your child's hearing is very precious. Some of the frequent causes of hearing loss are repeated ear infections, especially if they go untreated; maternal infections during pregnancy, such as rubella; certain medicines; and trauma to the ear. Permanent loss of high-frequency hearing can also occur with exposure to loud sounds. For example, rifle shots or gunfire can damage hearing, so earplugs are required at rifle ranges. A child may also be at risk if a substantial amount of time is spent listening to very loud music or television programs. Adolescents who prefer extremely loud music are at risk for high-frequency hearing loss.

Common Problems of the Outer Ear and Earlobe

Cuts and Bruises

The outer ear can be damaged by cuts or blows to the ear. Since there is such a rich blood supply to the area, it bruises and bleeds profusely when cut.

Pierced Ears

A child or even an infant may have pierced ears. They should be pierced by an experienced person so that trauma and chance of infection are minimized. It is best to use fourteen-karat gold posts, since most people do not suffer an adverse reaction to this metal. If your child does have a reaction, he or she may not be able to have pierced ears at this time, but you may wish to try the procedure again in the future.

Following piercing, the area around the earring should be cleaned two to three times daily with a cotton swab dipped in alcohol or hydrogen peroxide. The earring should be rotated gently so that any crust is removed. Before handling your child's ears, wash your hands carefully to minimize introduction of infection. The holes in the ears should be healed in about ten to fourteen days, and at that time the earrings may be removed for several hours without the holes closing. Be alert for signs of infection, such as redness, swelling, and drainage. If this occurs, remove the earring and apply a nonprescription antiseptic or antibiotic cream four times a day and clean the lobes with alcohol or hydrogen peroxide. If you are concerned or unsure about treatment, or if the infection does not improve or appears to worsen within forty-eight hours, contact your health care provider.

Foreign Objects

It is not unusual for the child under three to place a bean, pea, or other small object in the ear. The resulting symptoms may be vague and depend on the object placed there. It could cause pain, bleeding, or draining, especially if it deteriorates or causes an infection. Attempts at removing it may cause the object to perforate the eardrum, or you may harm the ear canal. Do not attempt to remove it yourself but see your health care provider. In some cases, objects have to be removed surgically.

Insects

Occasionally an insect can gain access to the ear canal. This causes pain and an intense noise from the movement of the insect. Do not attempt to remove the insect with a bobby pin or any other sharp instrument, or a cotton-tipped applicator. You could inadvertently damage the ear drum. The insect can be killed by placing oil ear drops in the ear and afterward irrigating the ear with water. Call your health care provider for instructions regarding ear irrigation. If the insect is not easily washed out, see your health care provider. If your child's eardrum is not intact or has polyethylene myringotomy tubes (commonly called P.E. tubes or simply tubes) in the eardrum, do not attempt to remove the insect by irrigation. Seek medical assistance because fluid can enter the middle ear through the tubes, possibly introducing an infection.

External Ear Infections

External ear infection, technically known as otitis externa, is an infection of the ear canal. It may occur in conjunction with a cold or as a result of a cut or of irritation of the lining of the ear canal, or because of frequent swimming. Your child can experience pain, itching, discharge from the ear, and possibly diminished hearing. The pain is intensified if you press on the ear directly in front of the opening to the ear canal above the earlobe. Generally, the presence of pain in this area distinguishes an external otitis from an internal otitis.

This condition needs treatment by a health care provider with prescription antibiotic eardrops and medication for the pain. Heat application to the external ear may also be prescribed.

Swimmer's Ear

Swimmer's ear is a type of external ear infection that commonly occurs when a child does a lot of swimming or diving. As the child swims, the ear canals are constantly immersed in water. The water flushes out the ear wax that protects the delicate lining of the ear canal. The skin of the canal becomes dry and itchy and may crack. Germs can enter this area and cause external ear canal infections. This disease can recur. Use of ear plugs when swimming helps to minimize recurrence.

Contact your health care provider before using nonprescription medicines, because the health care provider has the special equipment to visualize the ear canal and diagnose this condition.

Infections of the Middle Ear

It is estimated that as many as 80 percent of all children experience at least one ear infection by the time they reach adolescence. A middle ear infection, or otitis media, usually follows a cold, but it can occur following other childhood diseases such as measles, or even when the child appears otherwise healthy.

The short, straight eustachian tube of children under three years old appears to predispose them to infections. The young child also has little immunity to infections because of the lack of exposure to a large number of germs. In addition, some infants may drink from a bottle while lying on their backs. Remember that the opening to the middle ear, the eustachian tube, is in the back of the throat. When a child goes to bed with a bottle of juice or milk, fluid often pools in the back of the mouth. This provides an excellent culture medium for the growth of bacteria, and this bacteria can then move into the middle ear, where it can cause an infection.

Your child may complain of pain in the ear or pain upon swallowing when there is an otitis media. This is caused by a buildup of fluid or pus in the middle ear, which pushes on the eardrum, producing pain. The eustachian tube is closed, so the bacteria cannot escape, and if it continues to build up, it can rupture the eardrum. An infant exhibits ear pain by irritability, pulling on the ears, or banging his or her head on the side of the infected ear. Your child may or may not run a fever. With an otitis media it is not unusual for the temperature to range from normal to 104° F or higher.

Your child needs to be evaluated immediately by a health care provider, who will prescribe antibiotic therapy if an otitis media is present. A decongestant and a fever reducer may also be prescribed.

It is imperative that the medical treatment be followed as prescribed. The antibiotic needs to be taken for the full course of the therapy even if the child appears well after only a few days. The eardrum usually returns to normal in two weeks, with treatment. Many health care providers ask you to bring your child in for a reevaluation in ten days to three weeks following treatment of otitis media. It is important to keep this appointment, since the infection might still be present even though the child appears better. Lingering and recurring ear infections can damage a child's hearing.

Your child may develop several attacks of otitis media. Research indicates that a child under one year of age who has an otitis media is likely to experience another infection. Chronic otitis media occurs when the ear infection has failed to heal in response to an antibiotic. Your health care provider may first try other antibiotics; if this is unsuccessful, the placement of myringotomy tubes (P.E. tubes or simply tubes) in the eardrum may be inevitable. These are very small plastic tubes that prevent fluid from building up in the middle ear and thereby decrease infections for the child with a chronic problem.

Medicines for the Ear

Any child who has ear pain, drainage from the ear, hearing loss, or ringing in the ears should not be treated by nonprescription medicines but needs to be seen by a physician immediately. Since the eardrum cannot be visualized by the naked eye, it requires examination by a health care provider with an otoscope, an instrument that sends a narrow beam of light into the ear canal to aid visualization of the eardrum. As stated before, if the drum is ruptured or the child has P.E. tubes in place, it is especially important not to place any medicines or fluids into the ear, because the eardrum is not intact and germs can enter the middle ear, resulting in a middle ear infection.

Ear Wax Removal Medicines

Most authorities recommend that a child under twelve years not be treated with nonprescription ear wax removal agents. The child needs to be seen by a health care provider if excessive ear wax seems to be a problem.

Excessive ear wax causes a sensation of fullness in the ears or decreased hearing. Ear wax removal agents are designed only to soften the wax; they do not remove it. This must be done by water irrigation or by having a trained health care provider remove it manually. Do not attempt to irrigate your child's ear unless you have been instructed on how to do so by a health care provider. If the eardrum has been ruptured without your knowledge, you could cause damage by introducing water into the middle ear.

CARBAMIDE PEROXIDE 6.5% IN GLYCERIN

Trade Names: Benadyne Ear Drops Improved, Debrox, Murine Ear Drops.

Dosage Forms: Liquid eardrops.

Why Used: The carbamide peroxide loosens the debris and wax, and the glycerin softens the ear wax.

How to Give: Solution must remain in the canal for fifteen minutes. This is best accomplished by having your child remain on the side in the position in which you instilled the drops for fifteen minutes after the instillation. Do not allow your child's head to move. Irrigation is necessary for wax removal. Administer ear drops as directed for children over twelve in Chapter 4. Instill the number of drops as directed by the manufacturer.

Unintended Effects:

- Glycerin may irritate broken skin in the ear canal.
- If rash or local redness develops, it may indicate a sensitivity to the medicine. Discontinue use.

Contraindication: Previous allergy to this drug. Do not use if ear is draining or in an ear with myringotomy (P.E.) tubes in place. Do not use if ear canal is red, tender, or painful prior to administration without consulting your health care provider.

Special Note: If rash, local redness, pain, dizziness, or other adverse reactions occur, discontinue use of medicine and consult your health care provider. Use with caution to avoid getting this solution into the eyes.

Storage Instruction: Store at room temperature in a locked, secure medicine container out of reach of children.

Age Limitation: It is not recommended for use in children under twelve years.

Medicine for Swimmer's Ear

ALUMINUM ACETATE

Trade Name: Dri-Ear, Dumebro.

Dosage Forms: Liquid eardrops.

Why Used: It increases the acidity of the ear canal, creating an environment unfavorable for bacterial growth. It also toughens the skin of the ear canal and has a drying effect by reducing the secretory function of the skin glands.

How to Give: Administer ear drops as directed for children over twelve in Chapter 4. Instill the number of drops as directed by the manufacturer.

Unintended Effects:

- Rare with proper usage.
- Rash and local redness indicate a sensitivity to the medicine, in which case the medication should be discontinued.

Contraindication: Previous allergy to this drug. Do not use if ear is draining or in an ear with myringotomy (P.E.) tubes in place.

Special Notes:

- This substance should be prescribed by your health care provider, because the physician has the special equipment to visualize the ear canal and diagnose swimmer's ear.
- Discontinue if rash or local redness occur, and contact your health care provider.
- Use with caution to avoid getting this solution into the eyes.

Age Limitations: Seek advice from your health care provider before giving to a child under sixteen years.

Storage Instruction: Store at room temperature in a locked, secure medicine container out of reach of children.

CHAPTER 12

Medicines for Skin Disorders

Have you ever thought of the skin as a body organ? It is one of the largest and most important. It is through the skin that a large amount of sensory input occurs. This important function is experienced by an infant as you hold, cuddle, feed, tickle, bathe, and caress him or her. Through the sensations of touch as well as sight, hearing, and smell, your baby learns about the world and begins to trust people.

The skin also acts as a barrier to protect the body from harmful substances in the environment. It regulates the outward flow of water and electrolytes such as sodium and potassium, maintaining the delicate balance of body fluids necessary for life. The skin is able to regulate heat loss and retention, thus playing an important role in maintaining body temperature. Thus what at first appears to be a mere vessel for the body becomes a powerful, interactive, diversely functioning organ at closer inspection. Perhaps this explains why no one escapes without some skin problem during life, and why you undoubtedly have some questions about treatment of your child's skin rashes, dryness, or diseases. Understanding the different skin layers and their functions makes the explanations of skin disorders and treatments clearer.

The skin is a thin surface from 3 to 5 millimeters (about ⅛ inch) thick. It is composed of three layers. The outermost layer, called the epidermis, is thinnest and contains aging cells that are constantly being discarded from the skin surface, an area of actively dividing cells, and the melanin or pigment, which provides skin color.

The second layer, the dermis, contains the blood and lymph vessels, which bring nutrition and warmth to the skin cells. It is made up of many nerve endings and is therefore responsible for sensation. Hair originates in the dermis and is nourished by the rich blood supply of the area. The arrector pili muscles, those that make our hair stand up when we shiver, are in the dermis. Sweat glands secrete fluid to help regulate body temperature and are found both in the dermis and the lower, subcutaneous, skin layer. Sebaceous glands, also present in both areas, produce sebum, an oily substance that keeps the skin moist.

The innermost, or subcutaneous, skin layer contains additional blood vessels, sweat and sebaceous glands, and the fatty tissue that provides structure, elasticity, and heat regulation for the skin.

Common Skin Disorders

In Infancy

There are a number of reasons an infant experiences more and different skin ailments than an older child. The infant's skin is thin and

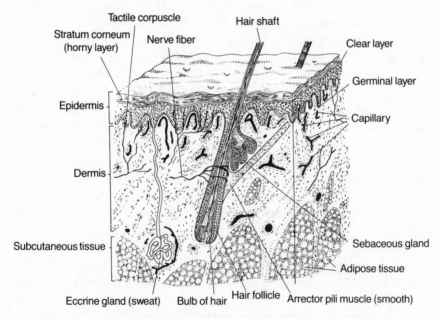

A cross section of the human skin. *(From Pansky, B., Dynamic Anatomy and Physiology, Macmillan, New York, p. 300.)*

has minimal secretion of sebum and sweat, which leads to frequent dryness. Due to its thinness and lack of oil, the skin's protective ability is therefore less, causing a greater number of rashes and other surface infections. In addition, the skin is less acidic than more mature skin, allowing bacteria to thrive more readily. The undeveloped immune system of the infant increases the incidence of many minor skin ailments, though antibodies acquired from the mother protect the infant from some communicable skin diseases in the early months of life. The thinness of the skin allows substances to penetrate into the body easily. For this reason harsh substances such as rubbing alcohol, hexachlorophene, Borax, or DMSO should not be applied to a baby's skin. These can be absorbed into the body and cause severe problems internally. Medicines applied to the skin of an adult or child should not be used on an infant before checking with a health care provider. In general, it is best to minimize the number of skin products used on infants.

The color of a baby's skin is usually different from that of adults. The thinner epidermis allows the blood flow in the dermis to become visible. Thus when a baby cries, the skin looks quite red, whereas when a baby is cold, a bluish tinge is noted in the hands and feet. This blueness is normal and changes as the baby moves around and becomes warmer.

Diaper Rash

Rash in the diaper area is experienced by nearly all infants at some time. It can be caused by a combination of factors. Sensitive skin, prolonged contact with urine or feces, or reactions to detergents, fabric softeners, plastics, or perfumes in diapers are the most common irritants.

Measures to treat diaper rash also help to prevent it. Don't delay in changing your baby's diaper as soon as it is wet or dirty; clean the area thoroughly with a baby wash product or plain water, and dry thoroughly. A thin application of ointment or powder can be used to protect the skin from urine and feces. Do not sprinkle powders (especially talcum powder) on the diaper area, since the small particles released into the air can be harmful when breathed into your baby's lungs. Instead, place the powder in your hand and gently pat it into place on the baby. Most of the diaper products available contain a substance to protect the skin; some also contain a product to retard growth of bacteria and fungi. Wash the product off and reapply it at each diaper change.

Expose the diaper area to air for at least twenty minutes daily when your baby has a rash. Place a waterproof pad on the floor or in the playpen or crib, cover it with a soft blanket or diaper, and let your baby lie on the surface without a diaper. Avoid plastic pants, since they prolong the contact of irritants with the skin. If you wash your own diapers, soak them in an antibacterial solution (such as ½ cup Borax in 1 gallon water), launder in mild soap, and rinse well with plain water. If you use a fabric softener, rinse the diapers again with plain water. If you change your brand of soap just before a diaper rash occurs, be suspicious of the new soap as the culprit.

When a diaper rash occurs it is important to treat it with vigorous action, since the dry, open skin it creates becomes a site for infection with bacteria or fungus. If the diaper rash continues for more than two to three weeks or spreads and worsens rapidly, contact your health care provider, since a prescription medicine may be needed.

Dry Skin

Due to immature sweat and sebaceous glands as well as the change from the protected and moist environment of the uterus to the dryer environment of the world, an infant's skin is often quite dry. If your baby has dry, flaking skin, minimize bathing with harsh soaps. A simple daily sponge bath with mild baby soap or plain water is all the baby needs. Make sure creases under arms, in groin, and in the neck and wrist areas are cleaned and dried thoroughly. A small amount of baby oil applied to dry areas can provide similar protection to that natural skin oil provides. Since dry, cracked skin allows infections to occur more easily, it is important to keep the skin clean of urine and feces. Providing humidity in the home, especially in dry winter months; drinking plenty of water daily; minimizing excess bathing; and using mild, oil-based soap can help prevent dryness at any age.

Cradle Cap

Flaking on the scalp is often due to a form of seborrhea. The first treatment is to rub the area well with a washcloth while cleaning with baby shampoo during the daily bath. If the condition continues after several days of such cleaning, rub the scalp with baby oil, leave it on for several hours, and then scrub gently with an antiseborrheic shampoo.

Prickly Heat

Red, raised, pimplelike rashes in skin creases often occur during warm weather and are the result of plugged sweat glands. The best solution is to avoid excess, tight, or restrictive clothing and to cover plastic car seats, crib mattresses, and the like with airy cotton covers. Clean areas of prickly heat with mild soap and water, dry thoroughly, and allow to remain open to air. Avoid application of ointments and powders, so the plugged sweat glands can breathe.

In addition there are a number of skin conditions that are normal during infancy and require no treatment. These include milia (small white spots on the face) and Mongolian spots (blue-gray patches across the buttocks). Check with your health care provider before treating any skin condition during infancy.

In Childhood

During early childhood the skin toughens and thickens, providing a stronger barrier to disease. The sweat glands are fully functional by early preschool age, while the sebaceous glands are not fully active until puberty. With the growing maturity of your child's skin, the irritant rashes of infancy are rarely seen in childhood. Instead, communicable diseases become more common as contact with other children increases. Skin injuries also occur as children become more active in play. The rashes of measles (rubeola) and German measles (rubella) are not discussed here. We encourage you to obtain immunization for these diseases when your child is about fifteen months of age so that they can be avoided. If you suspect your child has one of these communicable diseases, contact your health care provider for instructions.

Chickenpox

There is as yet no immunization approved for general use to prevent chickenpox, and thus the disease has to be treated by parents. Chickenpox is acquired by breathing in the virus of an infected person. Since it takes about two weeks to manifest itself, the infection is often transferred to many other children before the characteristic spots appear. Round, fluid-filled blisters are present on the head, in the mouth, and on the body, with the arms and legs, hands, and feet least affected. They eventually break open, "weep" fluid, and form a scab. The blisters are itchy, and treatment centers on relieving the itch so that scratching, infection, and scarring are avoided. Frequent baths in baking soda with slightly cool water can be used, and calamine lotion, a nonprescription drying agent, can be applied to the lesions. Put mittens over your child's hands during sleep to prevent scratching. Keep the nails short and clean. If the itching is excessive, contact your health care provider, since a prescription medicine may help. Prevent your child from contact with other children until all blisters have dried and scabbed; until this happens the disease is contagious.

Eczema

Eczema is a term used to describe a skin reaction that may be caused by contact with substances outside the body or by internal agents. The reaction involves redness and itching of skin, open fluid "weeping" of the area, and finally scaling, thickening, and altered pigmentation if the disease becomes chronic. Although eczema is not caused by fungus or bacteria, the open lesions can readily become infected, so frequent inspection for signs of impetigo or other infections is advisable.

Cleanse the area involved with tepid water; avoid harsh soaps; and add an oil to bath water to decrease dryness. Protection of the skin with medicated hydrocortisone or nonmedicated powder may be helpful. Medicated ointment or cream can be systemically absorbed, so it should be used for short periods and in small amounts unless directed otherwise by a health care provider. Avoid harsh detergents and soaps, excessive heat and dryness, bubble baths, wool and elastic clothing.

As foods can cause eczema in some children, you are encouraged to introduce infants to only one new food at a time. Citrus juices, eggs, wheat, corn, and cow's milk are common causes. If one of the child's parents has eczema or other allergic ailments (such as hay fever, asthma, or bee sting allergy), your child is more likely to develop eczema or another allergic illness. In this case extra attention to skin care and introduction of new foods are especially important.

Mild eczema is treated by the methods just described; more severe symptoms may require oral medicine such as antihistamines and corticosteroids and so require medical care. Any change in eczema should be evaluated by your health care provider.

Most infant eczema improves spontaneously by the time the child is two years old, so you can look forward to this. If eczema continues past that age, it is usually mild and occurs in areas such as creases in elbows, knees, and groin.

Head Lice

Suspect head lice, known as pediculosis, when your child scratches the head vigorously or has reddened areas behind the ears and along the neck. The eggs are visible as small white or gray substances that cling to the hair near the scalp. They look like flakes of dandruff but are not easily removed. By having your child hang the head down, you can look for these especially along the nape at the hairline. If you have questions, the school nurse or public health nurse is usually an expert in identifying head lice. Head lice are seen in children of all socioeconomic groups and with all states of cleanliness. Do not be embarrassed or ashamed if your child acquires head lice. Their presence is a result of contact with someone with the disease and not indicative of poor hygiene.

The disease is treated by nonprescription or prescription shampoo or lotion. After treatment, the dead nits, as the eggs are called, are then removed by combing the hair vigorously with a fine-toothed comb or rinsing with about a quart solution of half vinegar and half water. If you are certain of the diagnosis, you may choose to treat the child yourself. If you are uncertain or if the infection persists beyond the second shampooing or first lotion treatment, contact a health care provider.

Since head lice are easily transmitted by contact with infected items, treatment also needs to include the following: Clothing and bedding should be dry-cleaned or laundered in very hot water. Brushes and combs should be discarded or cleaned in boiling water. Sprays to kill lice are available in pharmacies for use on furniture and rugs. Check other family members and treat if necessary. Inform the teacher if your school-age child has head lice. All children in the class should be checked. Items that can transmit the disease in school should be appropriately cleaned. Teach your child not to lend or borrow combs. Schools should inform parents when head lice are found on a child so you can carefully inspect your own child's head.

Check your child within one week of treatment for further symptoms of lice and again check all family members to be sure the disease was not transmitted to them. A repeat treatment with antiparasitic shampoo is recommended seven to ten days after the first to kill newly hatched lice. A final word: Nearly all children will contract head lice sometime during childhood; close contact with other children makes this nearly unavoidable.

Impetigo

Impetigo is an infection of streptococcal or staphylococcal, commonly known as strep and staph, bacteria. It begins anywhere on the body, usually in an open skin area, and spreads readily to other body parts and other children. Insect bites, cuts, and dermatitis such as diaper rash are often the beginning sites for impetigo. Raised, reddened areas become pus-filled, "weeping" with liquid, and finally crust covered. Impetigo is caused by a bacteria, spreads rapidly, and requires treatment with an antibiotic. Contact your health care provider for diagnosis and a prescription, and keep your child home until the health care provider states that it is safe to return to school, day care, and other activities. The antibiotic may be applied to the skin, taken by mouth, or occasionally given by injection. Moisten and remove crusts with water before applying antibiotic ointment. Careful hand washing and clothing hygiene is needed to prevent further infection of your child and others. Keep your child from touching the sores, since this spreads the infection from one spot to another.

Poisonous Plants

Some persons exhibit a hypersensitivity reaction in response to plants. A substance in the plant acts as an antigen to provoke an antibody reaction in the sufferer, in the same way that hay fever is a hypersensitivity reaction caused by pollens in the air. Not all persons who come in contact with poison ivy, poison oak, or poison sumac show signs of reaction. Those who react begin to experience itching and redness on the part of the body that came in contact with the plant, most often hands or legs. The red areas often become raised and then fill with fluid. This fluid is not contagious. The rash is spread to other body parts when the antigen is transferred to them by touching the affected part. Careful washing and scrubbing immediately after contact with the plant minimizes spread. After about one week the irritation usually decreases on its own.

Treatment centers on relieving discomfort. Nonprescription preparations such as calamine lotion or hydrocortisone cream or prescription corticosteroids are used to decrease itching.

Immunity does not develop after the initial exposure. With each contact, symptoms reappear. Learning to identify and avoid the plant is the best prevention of future problems.

Ringworm

Tinea capitis and Tinea corpus are the technical names for ringworm of the scalp and body, respectively. It is caused by fungus and gets its name from the characteristic circular lesion of the skin, hair, or nails. The infection can be acquired from other infected persons, animals, or the soil. It can spread from one skin area to another in an infected child. Your child should be seen by a health care provider for diagnosis and treatment.

Ticks

Ticks are small insects that bury their heads in a child's body. Some of them transmit Rocky Mountain spotted fever, which can be a harmful disease. Ticks are often found on warm body parts such as the scalp, neck or waistline following camping or hiking. Cover the tick with salad oil, mineral oil, petroleum jelly, or alcohol and gently remove the tick with tweezers. Be sure no part of the tick remains embedded in the skin. Clean the area and your hands thoroughly with soap and water before and after treatment.

Rocky Mountain spotted fever occurs in a small number of persons following a tick bite. The disease occurs throughout the United States, not only in the West. One to eight days after being bitten, fever, loss of appetite, headache, rash beginning on the lower legs or arms, and restlessness may occur. See your health care provider if any of these symptoms become evident.

In Adolescence

The skin of the adolescent is like that of the adult. The increase in sebaceous gland activity during this period is due to changing hormone levels and leads to the common occurrence of acne. The increase of sebum, or oil, however, protects the adolescent from some of the common skin diseases of childhood.

Acne

Acne is an inflammation of the sebaceous glands as their activity increases in adolescence. Nearly all adolescents manifest some acne, while over half have cases severe enough to produce discomfort and require treatment. One of the major problems with acne is the emotional discomfort it causes. To a teenager, body appearance is very important, so pimples anywhere on the body can be intolerable.

Understanding the cause of acne may help your son or daughter cope with the condition. Due to hormone increase during adolescence, the sebaceous glands increase sebum production. Consequently the skin becomes more oily, and the ducts leading from the glands to the skin surface can become clogged, causing whiteheads or blackheads. An inflammation and minor infection in the blocked duct leads to the pimples.

Treatment centers on removing excess sebum from the body by frequent washing with simple soap, warm water, and washcloth as well as frequent hair shampooing. Avoidance of cosmetics and creams with oily ingredients is also recommended. Although avoidance of foods such as chocolate and colas is recommended by some, there is no conclusive evidence that diet worsens the inflammation. Several nonprescription products are available for skin cleansing. An oral antibiotic, usually tetracycline, and topical vitamin A are sometimes prescribed for long-term treatment of more severe cases.

Most acne ends spontaneously by the late teens or early twenties. The aim during the adolescent years is to manage the disease to minimize complications and scarring and to maintain a positive self-image.

Athlete's Foot

Athlete's foot is a fungus infection that causes peeling, tender, itching skin on the foot, particularly between the toes. The infection spreads from one person to another in showers and swimming pools. It is more frequent in warm, humid weather and when tight footwear without air circulation is worn. Wash the feet frequently and dry well. Use absorbent cotton socks and leave the feet open to air when possible. A nonprescription skin powder is often effective, but if the infection persists or spreads, see your health care provider.

Acne Medicines

BENZOYL PEROXIDE

Trade Names: Epi-Clear, Oxy 5, Parsadox, Vanoxide.

Drug Class: Keratolytic.

Dosage Forms: Gel, skin wash.

Why Used: For treatment of acne. It acts as a skin irritant, causing peeling of the outer, affected skin layer.

How to Give: The involved skin should be cleaned and the drug applied once or twice daily.

Unintended Effect: Allergic skin reaction may occur.

Contraindication: This drug should not be used if the adolescent has shown prior allergy to it.

Special Notes:

- For external use only.
- Avoid contact with eyes and mucous membranes (mouth, nose, genital region).
- This drug may bleach hair and fabrics.
- If acne persists and is troublesome, the adolescent should see a health care provider. There are prescription products that can be used for acne treatment.

Age Limitations: There is a lack of study of the effects of this drug on children, so it should only be used during adolescence or older ages unless directed otherwise by a health care provider.

Storage Instructions: Keep at room temperature with cover tightly closed.

SALICYLIC ACID

Trade Names: Listerex, Saligel Acne Gel. In addition, there are a number of products that combine salicylic acid with sulfur and/or other products. Trade names include Acno, Acnotex, Akne Drying, Acnaveen Cleansing Bar, Buf, Fostex Cake, Pernox.

Drug Class: Keratolytic.

Dosage Forms: Soap, lotion.

Why Used: For treatment of acne. It is believed to act as a skin irritant, causing peeling of the outer, affected skin layer.

How to Give: Apply to affected skin as directed on package label.

Unintended Effect: Excessive irritation of skin.

Contraindication: This drug should not be used if the adolescent has shown prior allergy to it.

Special Notes:

- For external use only.
- Salicylic acid is believed to be more effective when used in a combination product with sulfur than in the single ingredient form.
- Avoid contact with eyes and mucous membranes (mouth, nose, genital region).
- If acne persists and is troublesome, the adolescent should see a health care provider. There are prescription products that can be used for treatment.

Age Limitations: Use only in adolescence or older ages unless directed otherwise by a health care provider.

Storage Instructions: Keep at room temperature with cover tightly closed.

SULFUR

Trade Names: Acne Aid, Acnederm, Acnomead, Epi-Clear, Noxzema 12-Hour Acne Medicine, Transact. In addition, there are a number of products that combine sulfur and resorcinol. Trade names include Acne Aid, Acne-Dome, Acnomel, Clearasil, Exzit, pHiso Ac, Sulforcin.

Drug Class: Keratolytic.

Dosage Forms: Cream, liquid, cleanser, stick.

Why Used: For treatment of acne. It acts as a skin irritant, causing peeling of the outer, affected skin layer. It may also be effective against some of the microorganisms that cause acne.

How to Give: Apply to affected skin as directed on package label.

Unintended Effect: Excessive irritation of the skin.

Contraindication: This drug should not be used if the adolescent has shown prior allergy to it.

Special Notes:

- For external use only.
- Avoid contact with eyes and mucous membranes (mouth, nose, genital region).
- If acne persists and is troublesome, the adolescent should see a health care provider. There are prescription products that can be used for acne treatment.

Age Limitations: Use only in adolescence or older ages unless directed otherwise by a health care provider.

Storage Instructions: Keep at room temperature with cover tightly closed.

Antibiotics

There are several nonprescription antibiotics available for preventing and treating minor skin infections. These contain bacitracin, neomycin, polymixin, gramicidin, or tetracycline, singly or in various combinations.

Trade Names: Achromycin, Baciguent, Baximim, Furacin, Myciguent, Mycitracin, Neo-Polycin, Neosporin, Polycin, Polysporin, Spectrocin, Triple Antibiotic Ointment.

Drug Class: Antibiotic.

Dosage Form: Ointment.

Why Used: Antibiotics stop the growth of some bacteria, thereby preventing or treating the infection they cause.

How to Give: Clean the skin with mild soap and water and dry well. Use a clean or gloved finger or a clean piece of gauze or a tongue depressor to apply a thin layer of ointment to the affected skin.

Unintended Effects:

- Some persons are allergic to specific antibiotics. When they are administered to the skin, this allergy is shown by redness, blisters, itching, swelling, or burning.

Contraindication: Allergy to any of the antibiotics contained in the product.

Special Notes:

- For external use only.
- These antibiotic ointments may be used on minor new wounds to prevent infection. They are not recommended as effective for treating existing infections.
- Small skin infections are best treated by cleaning and soaks with warm water. If the infection worsens or is accompanied by pain, fever, or red streaks leading from it, see a health care provider.
- These medicines should not be put in the eye or applied to large areas of the body.
- Use these topical antibiotics for no more than one week; if the infection persists longer, see your health care provider.

Age Limitations: None.

Storage Instructions: Keep at room temperature with cover tightly closed.

Antiseptics

HYDROGEN PEROXIDE

Trade Names: Available as hydrogen peroxide.

Drug Class: Cleaning agent.

Dosage Form: Liquid.

Why Used: Cleanses drainage and debris from skin wounds.

How to Give: Apply to wound by pouring it directly or applying on a sterile gauze pad and allow to foam.

Unintended Effects: None known.

Contraindications: None.

Special Notes:

- For external use only.
- Hydrogen peroxide must be open to the air to be effective so should not be used on abscesses; neither should a bandage be applied immediately after use.
- If the skin wound is extensive, worsens, or is accompanied by pain, fever, or red streaks leading from it, see a health care provider.

Age Limitations: None.

Storage Instructions: Keep at room temperature in original dark bottle since it is light sensitive.

IODOPHORS

Trade Names: Betadine, Isodine, Poviderm.

Drug Class: Antiseptic.

Dosage Forms: Solution, ointment, sticks, and gauze pads.

Why Used: These complexes with iodine as the main active ingredient stop growth of some bacteria, thus preventing the infections they cause.

How to Give: Clean the affected skin with the iodophor preparation which has been placed on a sterile gauze pad, rinse with plain water, and dry well.

Unintended Effects: Is sometimes irritating to the skin.

Contraindication: Previous allergy to an iodine-containing preparation.

Special Notes:

- For external use only.
- May be used on new wounds to prevent infection. Not recommended as effective for treating existing infections.
- Small skin wounds are best treated by cleaning. If the wound is extensive, worsens, or is accompanied by pain, fever, or red streaks leading from it, see a health care provider.

Age Limitations: None.

Storage Instructions: Keep at room temperature with cover tightly closed.

MERBROMIN

Trade Name: Mercurochrome.

Drug Class: Antiseptic.

Dosage Form: Liquid.

Why Used: To clean small skin wounds and inhibit growth of germs.

How to Give: Clean area with soap and water first if dirty and apply the drug to affected area.

Unintended Effect: It can irritate the skin.

Contraindications:

- Previous allergy to mercury compounds.
- Do not use on large areas of raw or blistered skin, since it can be absorbed and act as a poison in the body.

Special Notes:

- For external use only. Do not use near the eyes.
- If fluid is escaping from the wound, the effectiveness of this drug on the bacteria present is decreased.
- If the wound is extensive, worsens, or is accompanied by pain, fever, or red streaks leading from it, see a health care provider.
- Mercurochrome is different from Mercurochrome II, which combines a different antiseptic (benzalkonium chloride) and two local anesthetics to decrease pain.

Age Limitations: None.

Storage Instructions: Keep at room temperature with cover tightly closed.

Medicines for Itching

CALAMINE

Trade Names: Caladryl (calamine with benadryl), Ivarest (calamine with benzocaine).

Drug Class: Drying agent.

Dosage Forms: Cream, lotion.

Why Used: To relieve itching caused by mild sunburn, insect bites, or contact with poisonous plants.

How to Give: Clean the skin prior to application. Shake the lotion and apply a thin layer of cream or lotion three to four times daily for no more than one week.

Unintended Effects: Burning or rash occasionally occur.

Contraindication: Do not apply calamine products to open or blistered skin.

Special Notes:

- For external use only.
- If the skin ailment persists or worsens, contact your health care provider.
- Avoid contact with the eyes or mucous membranes of the mouth, nose, and genital region.

Age Limitations: None.

Storage Instructions: Keep at room temperature with cover tightly closed.

Medicines for Parasitic Infections

PYRETHINS WITH PIPERONYL BUTOXIDE

Trade Names: A-200, R&C, Rid, Triplex.

Drug Class: Antiparasitic.

Dosage Form: Shampoo (liquid or gel).

Why Used: The combination of the drugs pyrethins and piperonyl butoxide is effective in killing lice (head, body, pubic).

How to Give: The shampoos are lathered, left on the affected body part for five to ten minutes, and rinsed off. A repeat shampoo is recommended in seven to ten days to kill newly hatched lice.

Unintended Effects: Skin irritation and rash can occur.

Contraindications:

- The child allergic to ragweed may be allergic to pyrethins also.
- Do not use on open, inflamed skin.

Special Notes:

- For external use only.
- Avoid contact with the eyes, since the medicine is irritating and can injure them.
- Infection with head lice is common in school-age children due to their close contact with one another and does not reflect a lack of cleanliness in the home.

- Hairbrushes, combs, and bedding should be washed in very hot water to prevent reinfection or spread to others.
- If lice continue to be present after two shampoos with this drug, contact a health care provider, since a prescription product may be needed to eliminate the infection.
- Notify the school nurse, teacher, or caretaker if your child gets lice. All children in the class or day-care center need to be examined.
- Check all family members for lice when your child becomes infected. Head lice are noted as small whitish flecks near the hair shaft, particularly along the neckline.

Age Limitations: None.

Storage Instructions: Keep at room temperature with cover tightly closed.

Medicines for Fungal Infections

MICONAZOLE

Trade Name: Micatin.

Drug Class: Antifungal.

Dosage Forms: Cream, powder (regular and aerosol), liquid aerosol.

Why Used: To treat fungal skin infections such as athlete's foot, jock itch, and ringworm.

How to Give: Wash and dry affected area. Apply to the affected skin by liberally brushing on the powder, rubbing on the cream, or spraying the aerosol in the morning and evening.

Unintended Effects: Rarely causes skin irritation.

Special Notes:

- For external use only.
- This product should be used as recommended until symptoms subside.
- If the infection worsens, spreads, or is not improved in two to four weeks, contact a health care provider. There is a prescription drug that can also be used to treat these infections if needed.
- Miconazole may be used on a regular basis to prevent athlete's foot in the child who frequently becomes infected.
- Wash clothing and bedding that come in contact with the fungal infection in hot water to prevent spreading.

Age Limitation: Do not apply to children under two years before consulting a health care provider.

Storage Instructions: Keep at room temperature.

TOLNAFTATE

Trade Names: Aftate, Tinactin.

Drug Class: Antifungal.

Dosage Forms: Cream, powder (regular and aerosol), liquid.

Why Used: To treat fungal skin infections such as athlete's foot, jock itch, and ringworm.

How to Give: Wash and dry infected area. Apply to the affected skin by liberally brushing on the powder or rubbing on the cream or liquid in the morning and evening.

Unintended Effects: Rarely causes skin irritation.

Special Notes:

- For external use only.
- This product should be used as recommended until symptoms subside.
- If the infection worsens, spreads, or is not improved in two to four weeks, contact a health care provider. There is a prescription drug that can also be used to treat these infections if needed.
- Tolnaftate may be used on a regular basis to prevent athlete's foot in the child who frequently becomes infected.
- Wash clothing and bedding that come in contact with the fungal infection in hot water to prevent spreading.

Age Limitation: Do not apply to children under two years before consulting a health care provider.

Storage Instructions: Keep at room temperature. The solution becomes solid in cold temperature but liquifies again when warmed.

UNDECLYENIC ACID

Trade Names: Cruex, Desenex, NP-27, Quinsana Plus.

Drug Class: Antifungal.

Dosage Forms: Powder (regular and aerosol), ointment, liquid, foam, soap, cream, shoe spray.

Why Used: To treat fungal skin infections such as athlete's foot, jock itch, and ringworm.

How to Give: Cleanse skin with soap and water and dry. Apply to the affected skin area as directed on package label morning and evening.

Unintended Effects: None known.

Special Notes:

- For external use only. Do not use near eyes.
- If the infection worsens, spreads, or is not improved in two to four weeks, contact a health care provider. There is a prescription drug that can also be used to treat these infections if needed.
- Wash clothing and bedding that come in contact with the fungal infection in hot water to prevent spreading.

Age Limitation: None.

Storage Instructions: Keep at room temperature with cover tightly closed.

Medicines for Inflammation

HYDROCORTISONE

Trade Names: Caldecort, Clinicort, Cortaid, Cortif, Hycort, and others.

Drug Class: Antiinflammatory.

Dosage Forms: Cream, lotion, ointment.

Why Used: To reduce the inflammation, redness, and itching of some skin disorders. It is useful for discomfort caused by insect bites, poisonous plants, or products such as detergents and cosmetics.

How to Give: Apply a light layer to the skin every few hours.

Unintended Effects: The amount of medicine in the nonprescription preparation is regulated so that the unintended effect of skin irritation is very rare.

Contraindication: Do not use on open skin.

Special Notes:

- For external use only.
- Do not apply this medicine to large surfaces of the body or use for longer

than a few days unless directed otherwise by a health care provider.

- Leave skin areas open to the air after application, since bandaging may increase the drug's absorption through the skin.
- If the skin disorder continues for more than seven days, worsens, or another skin ailment occurs, see your health care provider.
- Notify the health care provider if you have applied this medicine to the child's skin and then seek health care for any reason.

Age Limitation: Do not apply to a child under two years except with the advice of a health care provider.

Storage Instructions: Keep at room temperature with cover tightly closed.

Diaper Rash Products

CORNSTARCH

Trade Names: Cornstarch is available in combination with various other products. Some examples of combination products are Diaperene BP, Diapa-Care Baby Powder, Johnson & Johnson Cornstarch Baby Powder, Mexsana Medicated Powder.

Drug Class: Absorbent.

Dosage Form: Powder.

Why Used: To keep skin dry and minimize diaper rash.

How to Give: Wash and dry the diaper area. Place the powder in your hand far from your baby's head and then smooth onto the diaper area at each diaper change.

Unintended Effects: None known.

Contraindication: Do not apply to oozing rash.

Special Notes:

- A variety of factors contribute to diaper rash. Keep your baby clean and dry. Be alert for new cleaning agents, disposable diapers, or newly introduced foods as possible irritants.
- If a diaper rash continues for two to three weeks or spreads and worsens rapidly, see your health care provider.

Age Limitation: None.

Storage Instructions: Keep at room temperature.

PETROLATUM

Trade Name: Vaseline Pure Petroleum Jelly.

Drug Class: Skin protectant.

Dosage Form: Jelly.

Why Used: To provide a barrier against urine and other irritants, preventing or treating diaper rash.

How to Give: Wash and dry the diaper area. Apply daily at bedtime to prevent rash; apply three to four times daily to treat an existing rash.

Unintended Effects: None known.

Contraindication: Do not apply to an oozing rash.

Special Notes:

- A variety of factors contribute to diaper rash. Keep the child clean and dry. Be alert for new cleaning agents, disposable diapers, or newly introduced foods as possible irritants.
- If your baby's diaper rash continues for two to three weeks or spreads and worsens rapidly, see your health care provider.

Age Limitation: None.

Storage Instruction: Keep at room temperature.

TALC OR TALCUM POWDER

Trade Names: Talc is combined with other drugs; some of the combination products are Ammens Medicated Powder, Johnson & Johnson Medicated Powder, Johnson Baby Powder.

Drug Class: Absorbent.

Dosage Form: Powder.

Why Used: To keep skin dry and minimize diaper rash.

How to Give: Wash and dry the diaper area. Place the powder in your hand far from baby's head and then smooth onto the diaper area at each diaper change.

Unintended Effects: If inhaled, talcum powder can cause breathing difficulty which in rare cases even leads to death.

Contraindications:

- Do not use on an oozing rash.
- Avoid if your child is asthmatic or has other breathing difficulty.

Special Notes:

- Keep away from your baby's head. Avoid creating a puff of powder while applying, so the child does not inhale the talc.
- Keep containers closed and out of reach of young children.
- Consider using a nontalc powder, lotion, or cream to prevent and treat diaper rash instead of talc; thus the unintended effects can be avoided.
- A variety of factors contribute to diaper rash. Keep the baby clean and dry. Be alert for new cleaning agents, disposable diapers, or newly introduced foods as possible irritants.
- If a diaper rash continues for two to three weeks or spreads and worsens rapidly, see your health care provider.

Age Limitation: None.

Storage Instructions: Keep at room temperature with cover tightly closed to avoid accidental inhalation.

ZINC OXIDE

Trade Names: Zinc oxide is available alone or in combination with other ingredients. Some combination products are B-Balm, Bab-Eze, Balmex, Caldesene, Comfortine, Desitin, Johnson & Johnson Medicated Powder.

Drug Class: Skin protectant.

Dosage Forms: Cream, ointment, powder.

Why Used: To provide a barrier against urine and other irritants, preventing or treating diaper rash.

How to Give: Wash and dry the diaper area. Apply daily at bedtime to prevent rash; apply to diaper area three to four times daily to treat an existing rash.

Unintended Effects: None known.

Contraindication: Do not apply to an oozing rash.

Special Notes:

- A variety of factors contribute to diaper rash. Keep the baby clean and dry. Be alert for new cleaning agents, disposable diapers, or newly introduced foods as possible irritants.
- If a diaper rash continues for two to three weeks or spreads and worsens rapidly, see your health care provider.

Age Limitation: None.

Storage Instructions: Keep at room temperature.

Sunscreens

AMINOBENZOIC ACID (FORMERLY P-AMINOBENZOIC ACID OR PABA)

Trade Names: Pabagel, Pabanol, PreSun 8, Solar Cream. It is also available in combination with other sunscreen products and in some cosmetics. Examples of trade names include PreSun 15, RV Paba Stick.

Drug Class: Sunscreen.

Dosage Forms: Lotion, cream, gel.

Why Used: To absorb ultraviolet radiation, thus preventing sunburn and promoting suntan.

How to Give: Apply liberally to skin and lips exposed to the sun.

Unintended Effects: Allergic skin reaction after applying the product and being exposed to the sun has occurred rarely.

Contraindications:

- Any prior allergic skin reaction after applying this drug and being exposed to the sun.
- If your child has experienced a photosensitivity reaction to a thiazide diuretic, sulfonamide, sulfonylurea, furosemide, or carbonic anhydrase inhibitor, all of which are prescription drugs, do not use a sunscreen with aminobenzoic acid, aminobenzoate, methyl anthranilate, padimate A or O. These can also cause a photosensitivity reaction.

Special Notes:

- For external use only.
- Avoid contact with eyes and mouth.
- Each sunscreen has a skin protection factor (SPF) on the basis of its ability to block ultraviolet radiation. Children who tan well and burn minimally can use a product with SPF of 2 or 3. Those who tan gradually and burn sometimes should use a product with SPF of 4 or 5. Those who tan slightly and burn easily should use a product with SPF of at least 6 or 7. Those who always burn should use a product with SPF of 8 or above. Sunscreen products list the SPF on their labels.
- Apply this product two hours before sun exposure for best results. Although some products are more water resistant than others, it is best to reapply after your child has gone swimming or engaged in exercise and again after several hours of sun exposure.
- Discontinue use if skin irritation occurs.

Age Limitation: None.

Storage Instructions: Keep at room temperature.

OXYBENZONE OR DIOXYBENZONE

Trade Names: This product is usually combined with other sunscreens such as padimate or homosalate. Some combination products are Block Out, Chap Stick Sunblock 15, Coppertone Shade, Eclipse, Sundown.

Drug Class: Sunscreen.

Dosage Forms: Lotion, lip balm.

Why Used: To absorb ultraviolet radiation, thus preventing sunburn and promoting suntan.

How to Give: Apply liberally to skin and lips exposed to the sun.

Unintended Effect: Rare skin irritation.

Contraindications: Children sensitive to benzocaine, sulfonamides, aniline dyes, or PABA should not use this product.

Special Notes:

- For external use only.
- Avoid contact with eyes and mouth.
- Each sunscreen has a skin protection factor (SPF) on the basis of its

ability to block ultraviolet radiation. Children who tan well and burn minimally can use a product with SPF of 2 or 3. Those who tan gradually and burn sometimes should use a product with SPF of 4 or 5. Those who tan slightly and burn easily should use a product with SPF of at least 6 or 7. Those who always burn should use a product with SPF of 8 or above. Sunscreen products list the SPF on their labels.

• Although some products are more water resistant than others, it is best to reapply after your child has gone swimming or engaged in exercise, and again after several hours of sun exposure.

• Discontinue use if skin irritation occurs.

Age Limitation: None.

Storage Instructions: Keep at room temperature.

CHAPTER 13

Medicines for Weight Control

Overweight

Management of weight is nearly a national obsession. Many teenagers attempt to emulate popular models with extremely thin figures, and media advertisers equate beauty with thinness. However, a child whose weight is 20 percent over the ideal is considered obese. Consult with your child's health care provider to find out if your child's weight is in the recommended range.

Although excessive concentration on weight is not recommended, a healthy concern for remaining within recommended weight ranges is beneficial. This decreases many disease risks such as hypertension and diabetes and leads to an overall feeling of well-being. The importance of weight maintenance in early childhood is now recognized. No longer is the fat baby necessarily seen as the healthy baby, because there is evidence to show that the overweight child has a greater likelihood of being an overweight adult. If one parent is obese, the child is more likely to become obese also. If both parents are obese, the likelihood increases even more. And the negative effects of excess weight in adults, such as hypertension, can be identified in overweight children as well.

The components of good nutrition and regular physical activity play the major parts in weight management. Avoiding solid foods before four to six months of age helps prevent overweight in the infant and young child. A cornerstone can be laid for life when household snacks consist of fruit and vegetable sticks rather than chips, cookies, and candy and

213

when the daily routine includes physical activities such as walking rather than driving to a nearby store.

Growth patterns should be monitored during well-child visits throughout childhood. Height and weight should be roughly proportionate. For example, if height is in the tenth percentile, weight in the tenth to twenty-fifth percentile is expected.

If weight, diet, and activity are monitored from early life, adjustments can be made when necessary, and it is unlikely that a major effort to lose weight will be required. However, this is easier said than done, and treatment of overweight is often required. For the overweight child, medicines for weight loss are rarely recommended, since these can seriously affect the growth of bone and muscle. Instead a carefully regulated diet and activity program should be instituted to maintain the present weight until height catches up to weight.

This is also the best treatment with overweight older children, but many teens and preteens have ready access to and use nonprescription diet products. For that reason, appetite suppressants, bulk producers, and artificial sweeteners are explored in this chapter. Although they may be used by some teens, appetite suppressants and bulk producers should not be used by younger children except under the supervision of a health care provider. In addition, continual increases and decreases in weight are unhealthy, and ongoing problems with weight management are best helped by consultation with dietitians, nurses, or physicians. Group meetings for overweight teens are especially helpful in fostering weight management over long periods of time.

Underweight

Some children have difficulty maintaining an adequate weight. Whether the cause is an abnormally high metabolic rate, an absorption deficiency, or excess physical activity, these children require as much attention and dietary management as do those who are overweight. If underweight is accompanied by other symptoms such as weakness, fatigue, brittle hair and nails, or rapid heart rate, medical advice should be sought. Tests may demonstrate treatable conditions such as deficiency of an absorptive enzyme or an excess of thyroid. A sudden weight loss is also reason for seeking medical evaluation; this often accompanies serious illness even before other symptoms are apparent. Nutritional supplements that are high in calories may be used in the child who is underweight. They are not discussed in this chapter since the underweight child should be evaluated and treated by a health care provider.

Anorexia Nervosa and Bulimia

Another cause of underweight is anorexia nervosa. This disease is primarily seen in adolescent girls, but it may occur in older or younger females and males as well. The affected person has a great fear of obesity, even though he or she is actually underweight. About 25 percent of normal body weight may be lost, but the person still feels fat. Excessive physical activity, dieting, and medicines such as laxatives are often used to lose weight. Sometimes anorexia nervosa is combined with another disease, bulimia, or binging followed by induced vomiting. Bulimia can even occur without anorexia nervosa in a person of normal weight. Both these diseases are serious and require the care of a health professional. If you suspect that your child might be affected, contact your health care provider or an adolescent health service.

Medicines for Weight Control

PHENYLPROPANOLAMINE

Trade Names: Propadrine, Rhindecon. This medicine is also available in combination with other drugs. Some examples of combination products are Acutrim, Anorexin, Ayds AM/PM, Cenadex, Dexatrim, Diet-Trim, Odrinex, Spantrol, and Vita-Slim.

Drug Class: Appetite suppressant.

Dosage Forms: Tablet, capsule (regular and sustained release).

Why Used: Phenylpropanolamine has a stimulant effect on the brain's satiety center, leading to decreased appetite. Some authorities believe this medicine is only minimally effective in decreasing appetite.

How to Give: A dose of 25 to 50 mg can be taken before meals three times daily. Acutrim timed release tablets contain 75 mg, and one tablet is taken daily following breakfast.

Unintended Effects:
* Increased heart rate and increased blood pressure may occur.
* Restlessness, nervousness, insomnia, nausea, or nasal dryness are occasional unintended effects.

- The incidence of unintended effects increases if the recommended dose of 25 to 50 mg three times daily is exceeded.

Drug and Food Interactions: Adolescents taking prescription medicines for heart problems should contact a health care provider before taking phenylpropanolamine. They could be at risk for serious unintended effects on the heart.

Caffeine has some of the same unintended effects as phenylpropanolamine, namely restlessness, insomnia, and nervousness. When both these substances are used, the degree of unintended effects increases.

Contraindications:

- Do not take if there was a previous allergy to this drug.
- If nervousness, dizziness, or insomnia occur, discontinue use of the medicine.
- It should be taken only under the supervision of a health care provider if the adolescent has high blood pressure, heart disease, depression, diabetes, or thyroid disease, or is taking one of the class of prescription medicines known as monoamine oxidase inhibitors.

Special Notes:

- Many of the appetite suppressants combine phenylpropanolamine with caffeine, vitamins, or other products. Read labels carefully.
- Do not exceed the recommended dose. The drug has been shown to be effective for only relatively short periods of time, so it should be taken for a maximum of twelve weeks.
- This drug is present in some nonprescription decongestant products to reduce nasal congestion. It is also a common ingredient in some illicit street drugs known as speed.

Age Limitation: This drug should not be taken to facilitate weight loss in children younger than adolescence unless they are under the supervision of a health care provider.

Storage Instructions: Keep at room temperature.

BULK PRODUCERS

Trade Names: Diet-Aid, Fiberall, Metamucil, Melozets, Serutan.

Drug Class: Bulk producer.

Dosage Forms: Tablets, powder, granules.

Why Used: Bulk producers absorb fluid and become large masses in the stomach and intestines and are used to achieve a feeling of fullness. The bulk produced has a laxative effect as well. The active ingredient is usually methylcellulose or psyllium.

How to Give: Mix the medicine with liquid as directed on the package just prior to drinking it; it will thicken if allowed to sit. Drink at least 8 ounces of water with this medicine to prevent intestinal obstruction.

Unintended Effects: The laxative effect mentioned may be excessive, unnecessary, and unhealthy. Obstruction of the esophagus or intestines is a rare unintended effect. Drink extra water to prevent this.

Drug and Food Interactions: The possibility of obstruction increases when bulk producers are used at the same time as medicines like codeine or opiate-containing medicines, which decrease bowel movements.

Contraindications: Diarrhea or other stomach and intestinal problems are contraindications to the use of bulk producers.

Special Notes: There is no demonstrated proof that bulk producers help to decrease food intake because the substance leaves the stomach within thirty minutes.

Age Limitations: Do not use in children younger than adolescence unless directed by a health care provider.

Storage Instructions: Keep at room temperature in a dry area.

SACCHARIN

Trade Names: Sucaryl, Sweeta.

Drug Class: Artificial sweetener.

Dosage Forms: Tablet, liquid, powder.

Why Used: Saccharin provides a sweet taste without adding calories to the diet. It is frequently used in diet foods and drinks.

How to Give: Add to food needing sweetening.

Unintended Effects:

- Some persons complain of a metallic aftertaste caused by saccharin.
- Rats that are fed large amounts of saccharin over a long period of time

have an increased incidence of bladder tumors. It is unknown if this effect occurs in humans, so the Food and Drug Administration requires cautionary labeling of saccharin-containing products.

Drug and Food Interactions: None.

Contraindications: None.

Age Limitations: None.

Storage Instructions: Keep at room temperature.

ASPARTAME

Trade Name: Nutrasweet, Equal.

Drug Class: Artificial sweetener.

Why Used: Aspartame was approved as a table top sweetener in 1981 and a sweetener for carbonated beverages in 1983. It is used to provide a sweet taste with less calories than sugar and with minimal aftertaste.

How to Give: Add to food needing sweetening.

Unintended Effects: Although large amounts of aspartame are associated with brain changes and tumors in experimental animal studies, these effects have not been demonstrated in humans. Moderation in amount of intake is advisable.

Drug and Food Interactions: It loses sweetening ability if used in cooked foods.

Contraindication: Persons with the disease phenylketonuria (PKU) or those who must avoid protein foods should not take in aspartame, since it contains phenylalanine.

Special Note: Aspartame should not be used in foods that will be cooked or baked, since it loses its sweetness when heated.

Age Limitation: None.

Storage Instructions: Keep at room temperature or cooled. Do not heat.

CHAPTER 14

Medicines for Menstrual Discomfort

Menstruation is one of several signs of puberty, the onset of which occurs somewhere between nine to sixteen years. The age at which menarche, the first menstruation, appears varies with each child and is influenced by heredity, race, state of nutrition, environment, and climate. Recently it has been found that young women involved in strenuous exercise programs may experience a delay in menarche. Researchers feel that this delay may be due to the ratio of lean body mass to body fat, a relationship that influences the hormonal regulation system.

Body Changes Associated with Puberty

Puberty is a developmental process and does not occur as a single event. When puberty begins in your daughter, you will notice several changes. Again, their appearance and onset vary from child to child.

Breast development is one of the first signs of puberty to appear in the female. Usually it starts with the nipple area becoming more prominent, caused by a small amount of tissue developing under each nipple. These are commonly called breast buds or budding of the nipples. Occasionally one breast starts to develop first, but within several months both nipples will be involved. The breasts increase in size, and a darkening of the areola or area surrounding the nipple occurs. These breast changes happen over a three- to four-year period. During the first two years your daughter will experience a growth in the bony pelvis, usually followed by an increase in skeletal height, a growth spurt. During

219

this time most girls gain a softening of the figure due to the increase in fat layers about the hips, arms, and chest region. At about the same time pubic hair begins to grow, and it will continue to increase until puberty is completed. Axillary (underarm) hair develops about two years after the beginning of the appearance of pubic hair. There are also internal changes occurring in the vaginal lining as well as external changes in the genitals. A deepening of the voice usually occurs, and acne may also develop during puberty. Menarche occurs about midway or toward the end of these body changes.

The hormones that trigger all these body changes also affect your daughter's moods. The hormonal changes, combined with the adjustment to the physical changes in the body, can be emotionally unsettling. Puberty is especially difficult for the young girl who lacks self-confidence. Research has demonstrated that early-maturing girls may be extremely stressed. The average school-age girl is developmentally ahead of the average school-age boy. The physically maturing young girl of eight or nine may feel conspicuous and out of place among her peers. This girl may respond by choosing to be with older children.

From all these changes you can see the need for understanding and sensitive parental support. Girls need factual information to help them understand what is happening to them. If it is difficult to discuss this topic with your daughter, contact your health care provider so information can be given to assist you, or someone else who is qualified can discuss the subject with her.

The Menarche

Anatomy of the Female Reproductive System

The female reproductive system is made up of the external genitalia and internal organs. These are present at birth and grow, mature, and change as puberty is experienced.

External Genitalia

The external female organs are often referred to as the genitalia or perineum. The fleshy thick folds of outer skin are called the labia majora. These two folds are covered with hair after puberty. When these are spread, the smaller, shorter folds of the labia minora become visible. They are shiny and look like mucous membranes. Inside this area at the upper fold region is the clitoris, and directly below is the urethral opening. This is the external opening of the tube that leads to the bladder where urine is held until urination. Directly below the urethra is the opening to the vagina. Just outside the folds of skin below the vagina is the rectal sphincter or the anal opening.

Internal Organs

The vagina is a muscular tube covered with a mucosal lining that continually rejuvenates itself. This is where the penis enters the female body during intercourse and is also the canal through which a baby is born.

At the internal end of the vagina is a strong set of muscles shaped

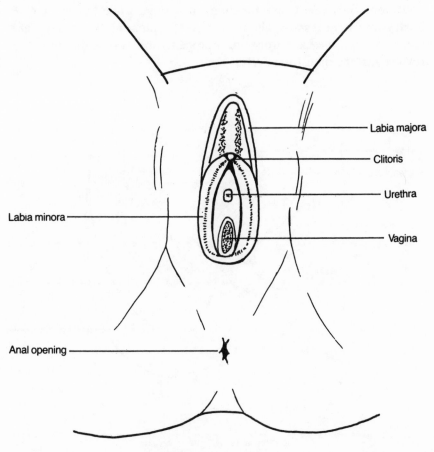

External female genitalia.

in a circular fashion, known as the cervix. It is smooth to the touch. The cervix closes off the womb, or uterus, from the vagina. It dilates during childbirth to allow the baby to be born.

The womb or uterus is a pear-shape organ about the size of a clenched fist. It is narrow at the cervical base and larger at the top. It is suspended by strong ligaments so it rests slightly forward and directly over the bladder. The uterus is composed of several layers of muscles and has a mucous membrane lining called the endometrium.

The fallopian tubes are two small tubes that arise from either side of the upper uterus and lead to the ovaries. These tubes enclose small, hairlike structures that function to move the ovum (the egg), from the ovary to the uterus, where it is deposited on the endometrium.

The two ovaries are located on each side of the uterus in the lower abdominal region. The ovaries function to release an ovum during ovulation. Only one ovary functions at a time, while the other rests. Each ovum is very small; about the size of a pinhead. The ovaries also secrete and synthesize estrogen and progesterone, two of the hormones involved in the menstrual cycle.

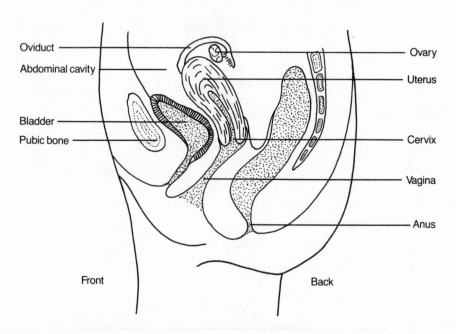

The internal female pelvic organs.

Your daughter is born with these internal organs and also with the total number of eggs her body will possess for the rest of her life. These organs are immature initially, but at puberty they become functionally mature.

Menstruation

Menstruation is not simply a process of the reproductive organs. It also involves the nervous and endocrine, or hormonal, systems of the body, which directly influence and regulate the reproductive organs.

Puberty begins when a gland in the brain, called the hypothalamus, stimulates the pituitary gland, also located in the brain, to release an increase in the hormone gonadotropin. Gonadotropin stimulates the ovary to secrete estrogen, which is responsible for many of the bodily changes seen in puberty. To more fully understand the menstrual cycle, one must look at the hormones involved and their effects on a girl's body.

Menses is really nature's way of ridding the body of products not used for pregnancy. Menstrual flow contains the broken-down endometrial lining of the uterus, which is composed of blood, cellular debris, mucus, and the unfertilized egg. With each period about 2 to 3 ounces (60 to 90 cc) of blood are lost, although the amount of blood loss varies from female to female. Some females may lose 6 to 7 ounces of blood. The amount of flow also varies with the female herself and with age. The average completely saturated pad or tampon absorbs about 1 ounce (20 to 30 ml) of fluid.

The menstrual flow is dark red in color and has an odor, most of which probably comes from decomposing blood cells. Each period of flow usually lasts from three to seven days, but it can be between two to nine days and still be considered normal. The average menstrual cycle is twenty-seven to thirty-one days, but it may be as long as forty days in some females. Each female has an individual cycle regulated by her hormone levels.

Menses in your daughter may be irregular at first, but there is no reason for concern because this is considered normal. It is important to realize that even though the cycle is irregular, pregnancy can still occur. If irregularity continues into the later teen years, consult your health care provider.

The hormonal cycle is nature's way of preparing the body for pregnancy. For discussion purposes, a twenty-eight-day cycle is used.

Day 1 of the menstrual cycle is the first day the flow starts.

The menstrual cycle is interdependent on the stimulation of the hypothalamus, the front (anterior) portion of the pituitary gland, the ovaries, and the uterus. During the first several days of the cycle the hypothalamus secretes a hormone that acts upon the pituitary. The pituitary gland secretes six hormones, three of which influence reproduction and two of which exert control over the menstrual cycle. These two hormones are the follicle stimulation hormone (FSH) and the luteinizing hormone (LH).

FSH stimulates a follicle in the ovary, which consists of an immature ovum and some tissue cells surrounding it, to start to mature. It also induces the ovary to produce estrogen, which, among other things, causes some females' breasts to become a bit larger and tender during the week just prior to the menses. Estrogen also causes the endometrium to thicken to six or eight times its original size, in preparation for the fertilized egg. This entire process is completed by midcycle, or the fourteenth day of a twenty-eight-day cycle. This is the time the body is considered to be fertile.

The increase in estrogen produced by the ovary stimulates the pituitary to produce LH. This hormone signals the mature follicle to rupture and release the ovum into the fallopian tube.

Some females experience pelvic discomfort during the period of ovulation. It may result from a small amount of blood entering the abdominal cavity when the ovum is released. This is called mittelschmerz.

During this midcycle phase the ovary also produces progesterone. The ruptured follicle becomes the corpus luteum, a yellow glandular mass left where the ovum was discharged from the follicle, that releases large amounts of progesterone. The progesterone causes the endometrium to double in thickness and become more spongy. Progesterone also stimulates the breasts to enlarge slightly and become more sensitive to touch.

Toward the end of the cycle the level of progesterone decreases if fertilization of the ovum and pregnancy have not occurred. The LH level decreases, which causes the endometrium to break down and the menses to begin. Then the cycle begins all over again.

Menstrual Problems

Lack of menstruation is called amenorrhea. If your daughter fails to menstruate by eighteen years of age or if the menses should stop for longer than three months, an evaluation by a health care provider is

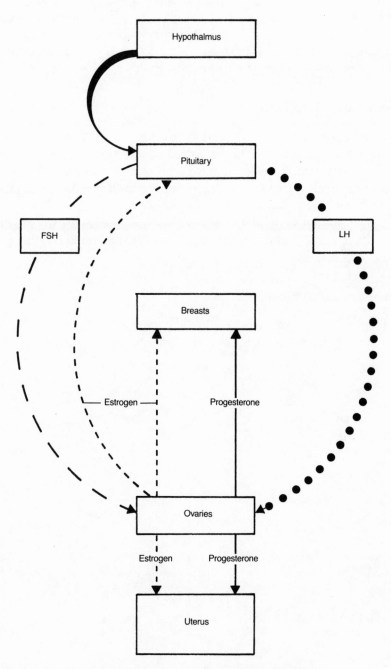

The female hormones and the organs they influence.

called for. There are many reasons that this may happen, most of which
are hormonal or genetic. Factors that may cause the menses to cease
once it has begun are also numerous, including severe weight loss,
pregnancy, and hormonal imbalance. Any girl who ceases to menstruate
needs to be seen as soon as possible by a health care provider.

Painful Menstruation

Painful menstruation is called dysmenorrhea. The nature of the
discomfort varies, but it is characterized by cramplike symptoms that
last for the first one or two days of the menses. Some women experience
severe cramplike symptoms, accompanied by headache, dizziness, upset
stomach, and loose stools.

If the symptoms are mild, nonprescription analgesics usually provide
adequate relief. If your daughter's pain is severe she should be evaluated
by a health care provider.

Premenstrual Syndrome

Premenstrual syndrome (PMS) is comprised of a collection of
symptoms that usually occur two to three days prior to the onset of

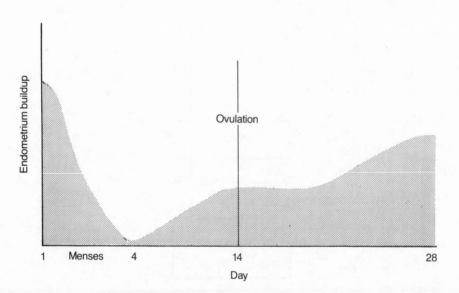

A schematic diagram showing the 28-day menstrual cycle.

menses or at the end. The exact cause is usually unknown. Most women complain of swelling of the ankles, feet, and/or face, sometimes with breast tenderness, headache, and weight gain, usually of less than five pounds. Other symptoms include abdominal fullness, constipation, feelings of depression, irritability, crying spells, and sleep disturbance. Some women have cravings for sweet or salty foods. If your daughter suffers from these symptoms, consult your health care provider.

Toxic Shock Syndrome

In 1980 toxic shock syndrome, or TSS, affected some tampon users who were otherwise healthy females. It occurred most frequently in women who used superabsorbent tampons. A specific type of germ, staphyloccous aureus, which is normally found on the skin or vaginal area, appears to start the disease process. Although the exact mechanism is not known, it seems the germ enters the body through the vaginal mucosa, it produces a by-product known as a toxin, which causes the symptoms: a fever of 102° F or higher, a sunburnlike rash on the palms of the hands and soles of the feet, which peels and sheds scales of skin, and a drop in blood pressure. There may also be upset stomach, diarrhea, sore throat, bruising or bleeding from any part of the body, lack of urination, and painful muscles. The appearance of these symptoms requires immediate medical care.

Vaginal Products

Feminine Hygiene Sprays

These are aerosol sprays designed to disguise perineal odor. The sprays do not contain medicinal ingredients and possess no therapeutic properties. The effect of these sprays is questionable, according to medical opinion. However, if a spray is used, follow the directions for frequency and method of application.

Sprays have been associated with irritation of the sensitive perineal area, itching, and swelling of the vagina. Read the label carefully for contents to notice any substance to which your daughter is allergic. Feminine sprays often contain perfumes for deodorant activity. Benzalkonium, benzethonium chloride, hexachlorophene, and chloroxylenol are chemical preservatives that do not kill bacteria. The propellent contained in the spray can cause local irritation to the genitals if the aerosol is applied too close to the perineum. All these properties can cause vaginal irritation leading to local swelling and itching. Sprays may also mask the odor from a vaginal infection, thus delaying its recognition and treatment.

Daily hygiene with soap and water are effective and sufficient for reducing perineal odor. However, care must be taken because deodorant soap can be sensitizing, too. Use only mild soap, and rinse the perineal area well.

Vaginal Douches

Many health care providers feel the vagina cleans itself by its natural discharge. If the external genitalia are kept clean with soap and water, odor is diminished. Normal vaginal health is dependent upon an acidic environment and a bacterial balance. If this balance is disturbed it may permit the vagina to become susceptible to infection. For example, if you daughter douches with a product that makes the vaginal area less acidic, it may permit certain types of bacteria already present to overgrow, because the conditions are more favorable for their growth, resulting in a vaginal infection. Some health care providers feel that douching, if done correctly and with the right solution, is not harmful. For your teenage daughter, it is best to consult with your health care provider for advice. Usually most teenagers do not need to douche. Girls need to know that douching does not prevent pregnancy. If your daughter has a vaginal infection, do not attempt to treat it by douching but consult your health care provider.

Sanitary Napkins

Sanitary napkins come in many sizes and shapes, from thin panty liners to thick absorbent pads. Your daughter should try several different types until she finds the brand that meets her needs. Some brands of teen and junior pads are designed for a young girl's smaller body. Deodorant napkins may cause a local reaction if your daughter is allergic to the perfume in the pad. Pads should be changed every two to six hours, depending on the amount of flow. This helps to reduce odor. Washing of the perineal area promotes hygiene and comfort. Teenagers are susceptible to advertising claims that a certain brand can make the user fresh and appealing. Your daughter can use your assistance in making these decisions.

Tampons

It is safe for teenagers to wear tampons if they have proper instructions on how to insert them. Tampons are made of absorbent cellulose and other manufactured materials. They do allow more freedom in sports and swimming than napkins. However, deodorant tampons may cause irritation or allergic reactions. If this should occur, discontinue use.

If a tampon is to be used, precautions against possible toxic shock syndrome must be taken. It is recommended that tampons be changed four to six times per day and used alternately with pads, such as using tampons during the day and pads at night.

Medications for Menstrual Discomfort

If your daughter has severe menstrual discomfort or other problems, she should be evaluated by a health care provider. For mild discomfort, one of the following medicines may help.

Analgesics

Some of the best medicines for mild menstrual cramps are the analgesic products of acetaminophen and aspirin. These products are probably less costly than those designed specifically for relief of menstrual discomfort. Ibuprofen, formerly a prescription medicine, is now available without a prescription. It is widely accepted as an effective agent for menstrual cramps.

ACETAMINOPHEN

Trade Names: Aspirin Free Anacin, Bromo-Seltzer, Co-Tylenol, Datril, Excedrin, Liquiprin, Panadol, Phenaphen, Tempra, Tylenol.

Dosage Forms: Tablets (regular and chewable), drops, elixer.

Why Used: Acetaminophen is an analgesic that reduces mild to moderate pain and an antipyretic that reduces fever. Its potency and action are similar to that of aspirin.

How to Give: Take as directed by manufacturer by mouth.

Unintended Effects: Acetaminophen is generally believed to have no side effects when taken in recommended dosages.

Contraindications: Acetaminophen is contraindicated in a child with liver disease and the rare child who shows hypersensitivity to this medicine.

Special Notes:

- There are two forms of liquid acetaminophen. One is an elixir and contains 120 mg of medicine in 5 ml of liquid, while the other is in the form of drops and contains 60 mg in 0.6 ml of liquid. Read labels carefully to avoid administering an incorrect dosage of medicine.
- The drug is broken down by the liver, so it can accumulate to toxic levels if given to a child with liver disease.
- Acetaminophen is combined with other drugs such as aspirin by some manufacturers. These products are usually more expensive and have not been shown to be more effective than the single-ingredient preparation.
- The drug is harmful if taken in excess. Keep it locked out of reach of children, and contact the Poison Control Center immediately if your child takes an excessive dose.

Age Limitations: Anacin is not recommended in children under six. Do not use Datril in children under twelve except under direct medical supervision. Do not use maximum strength or extra strength formulas in children under twelve years.

ASPIRIN (ACETYLSALICYLIC ACID)

Trade Names: Alka-Seltzer, Anacin, A.S.A., Ascriptin, Aspergum, Bufferin, Ecotrin, Encaprin, Empirin.

Dosage Forms: Tablet (regular, effervescent, enteric coated, chewable, and time release), rectal suppository, chewing gum.

Why Used: Aspirin is a salicylate product, which is effective as an analgesic to reduce mild to moderate pain, as an antipyretic to reduce fever, and as an antiinflammatory to reduce swelling and discomfort.

How to Give: Take as directed by manufacturer by mouth.

Unintended Effects:

- Aspirin commonly causes stomach distress, burning, nausea, and vomiting; more rarely, bleeding and ulcers.
- Aspirin alters the platelets of the blood, increasing the chances of bleeding throughout the body. The newborn baby's ability to clot blood is affected if the mother takes aspirin in late pregnancy.

- Occasionally children are allergic to aspirin, showing rash or breathing difficulty.
- When repeated doses are taken for long periods of time, aspirin can build up in the body. Symptoms of overdose in such cases are labored breathing, ringing in the ears, headache, stomach distress, bleeding, and agitation. Overdosage with aspirin remains a major source of poisoning for children. This medicine is powerful when taken in excess, causing serious illness and even death. Therefore, purchase aspirin in child-resistant containers and keep it locked out of your child's reach.
- An increase in numbers of cases of Reye's syndrome, a neurological disease, has been noted when young children are treated with aspirin for chickenpox or influenza. In the child with one of these problems, acetaminophen should be given rather than aspirin.

Drug and Food Interactions: Effervescent aspirin (e.g., Alka-Seltzer) is high in sodium, an important factor to consider if a child is on a low-sodium diet.

Aspirin interacts adversely with a number of prescription drugs that are infrequently administered in childhood. However, if your child is taking any prescription medicine(s) or large doses of vitamin C, check with your health care provider before administering aspirin.

Contraindications: Aspirin is contraindicated in persons hypersensitive to the medicine, in young children being treated for chickenpox or influenza, in late pregnancy, in those undergoing oral procedures (e.g., tonsillectomy or dental work), and in persons with bleeding disorders or kidney disease. Since it is excreted in breast milk, the nursing mother should minimize its use although an occasional dose should not harm the nursing baby.

Special Notes:

- Buffered aspirin is a special preparation that helps decrease the stomach irritation common with this medicine. The same effect can be created by administering aspirin with a glass of milk or other snack and is considerably less expensive than purchasing buffered or enteric-coated aspirin.
- Generic aspirin has not been shown to be less effective than trade brands and thus can be safely and effectively used.
- Time-release preparations have not been demonstrated to provide longer duration of action; neither do they minimize unintended effects. Their absorption is quite variable.
- Aspirin is available in combination preparations with other products such as caffeine. The effectiveness of these products has not been demonstrated,

and the resulting combinations are often much more expensive than aspirin alone. Read labels carefully.

- Aspirin dosage is often labeled in grains (gr), and since 1 grain is the same as 60 to 65 milligrams (mg), the adult aspirin tablets commonly used each contain 5 gr or 325 mg. Children's aspirin is available in 1 gr (60 mg), and 1¼ gr (80 mg) tablets.
- Rectal suppositories can irritate the lining of the rectum, and their absorption may be unpredictable, so tablets are recommended unless your child is vomiting. Tablets can be crushed and administered with a small amount of food for easy swallowing. Children's chewable tablets are also available.
- The chewing gum with aspirin (Aspergum) is often irritating to the inside of the mouth. If this should occur, discontinue use. Aspirin tablets will be just as effective, even to treat discomfort in the throat.

Age Limitations: Anacin is not recommended in children under six years. Do not use maximum strength or extra strength formulas in children under twelve years. Do not use arthritis formulas in children. Do not use Ecotrin in children under twelve years.

IBUPROFEN

Trade Names: Advil, Nuprin.

Dosage Form: Tablet.

Why Used: Ibuprofen is used as an analgesic to reduce mild to moderate pain and to decrease the swelling of inflammation. It also helps to reduce fever. Potency and action are similar to aspirin.

Unintended Effects: Upset stomach or heartburn may occur.

Contraindications: Do not give if your child has been hypersensitive to other nonprescription pain relievers. It is also contraindicated in late pregnancy, and should be taken only with advice of your health care provider if your child takes any prescription medicine.

Special Notes:

- This drug has been available by prescription and recently was approved for nonprescription use. It has not been widely tested in young children yet; thus the caution not to administer to children under twelve years.
- If the painful area becomes increasingly swollen or red, see a health care provider.

- This drug should not be taken at the same time as aspirin or acetaminophen unless directed to do so by your health care provider.
- Keep this drug locked out of reach of your children.

Age Limitations: Do not give this drug to children under twelve years without the advice of a health care provider.

Diuretics

Some women experience mild fluid retention just prior to their menses. This fluid causes irritability and pain. These symptoms are usually seen with premenstrual syndrome. Diuretics are drugs that act upon the kidneys or other organs to eliminate the excess water that has accumulated in the body. The following are mild diuretics used in the most common menstrual combination products.

AMMONIUM CHLORIDE

Trade Names: Ammonium chloride, ammonium chloride combination with other drugs, Aqu-Ban.

Dosage Forms: Tablets.

Why Used: It temporarily alters the body's salt and water ratio regulation by the kidneys. However, its effect is of short duration (one or two days).

How to Give: Take as directed by manufacturer by mouth. Do not use longer than ten consecutive days.

Unintended Effects: Doses of ammonium chloride of above 4 to 8 grams may cause upset stomach, vomiting, headache, dizziness, sleepiness, mental confusion, and increased respiration.

Contraindications: Do not give this medicine to a child with hypertension, heart disease, impaired liver or kidney function.

Age Limitations: Do not use in children under twelve years.

Storage Instruction: Store at room temperature in a locked, secure medicine container out of reach of children.

CAFFEINE

Trade Name: As a single-ingredient product, Tri-Aqua. Caffeine is also used in combination with other drugs. Some combination products are: Aqu-Ban, Flowaway Water 100's, Midol, Odrinil.

Dosage Form: Tablets, capsules, caplets.

Why Used: The medicines contain caffeine alone or in combination with other compounds. Caffeine is a mild diuretic. Some manufacturers claim that caffeine enhances the effect of analgesics when used in conjunction with them, and it may also help alleviate fatigue due to water retention. Such claims are questionable.

How to Give: Take as directed by manufacturer by mouth. Do not use longer than ten consecutive days.

Unintended Effects: Caffeine may cause stomach upset or irritability.

Contraindications: Individuals on a caffeine-free diet and persons with a sensitivity to caffeine should not take it.

Drug and Food Interactions: Coffee, tea, some sodas, and chocolate also contain caffeine and may enhance the unintended effects of caffeine if taken concurrently with a caffeine-containing medicine. The same amount of caffeine found in most medicines can be obtained by drinking a cup of coffee or a twelve-ounce can of caffeine-containing soda.

Special Notes: Read labels carefully to assess the properties of other drugs present in the medicine.

Age Limitations: Do not use in children under twelve years.

Storage Instruction: Store at room temperature in a locked, secure medicine container out of reach of children.

PAMABROM

Trade Names: Pamabrom is available in combination with other drugs, such as acetaminophen, aspirin, and antihistamines. Cardui, Pamprin, Sunril, and Trendar.

Dosage Form: Tablet, capsules.

Why Used: A mild diuretic that increases urinary output initially, pamabrom does not reduce swelling. In combination with analgesics and antihistamines, it reduces cramps, tension, and depressed feelings.

How to Give: Take as directed by manufacturer by mouth. Do not use longer than ten consecutive days.

Unintended Effect: Rare.

Contraindication: Do not take if sensitive to analgesics or antihistamines.

Special Notes:

- These drugs are in combination with aspirin or acetaminophen, so read the labels carefully before taking aspirin or acetaminophen concurrently. Do not take these drugs with antihistamines or diuretics, both prescription and nonprescription, before consulting your health care provider.
- Do not exceed 200 mg per day. Follow manufacturer's recommendations for administration.

Age Limitations: Do not use in children under twelve years.

Storage Instruction: Store at room temperature in a locked, secure medicine container out of reach of children.

Miscellaneous Ingredients

Based on clinical data, ingredients found in some combinations of natural herbs, such as buchu, uva ursi, mays, and couch grass, have a questionable diuretic efficacy.

Antihistamines

PYRILAMINE MALEATE

Trade Names: Cardui, Pamprin, Sunril.

Dosage Form: Tablet.

Why Used: Manufacturers claim that the medication blocks the release of histamines, which are present at an increased level at the start of menstruation. The efficacy of such action is uncertain, but it does have mild numbing and painkilling effects. Also its sedative properties may relieve depression and tension.

How to Give: Take as directed by manufacturer by mouth. Do not use longer than ten consecutive days.

Unintended Effect: Drowsiness common.

Special Note: Do not exceed 200 mg in any one day. These drugs are in combination with aspirin or acetaminophen, so read the labels carefully before taking aspirin or acetaminophen concurrently. Do not take these drugs with antihistamines or diuretics, both prescription and nonprescription, before consulting your health care provider.

Age Limitations: Do not use in children under twelve years.

Storage Instruction: Store at room temperature in a locked, secure medicine container out of reach of children.

Vitamins

Vitamin B_6 has been found effective in the treatment of premenstrual syndrome in subjects who are deficient in this vitamin. Its effectiveness in treating menstrual problems in general, however, is not well founded or proved.

PART FOUR

Common Prescription Medicines

The next three chapters describe medicines that are commonly prescribed for oral use in children. These are organized alphabetically in three pharmacological classes: medicines for infections, medicines for seizure and behavioral control, and medicines for the heart and lungs.

Information not included in these chapters are Recommended Dosages and Age Limitation. This is because the correct dosage of a drug has to be tailored for each child on the basis of age, body weight, illness, and physiological conditions. If you have any questions concerning dosage of a drug, contact the prescriber.

Age Limitation on the use of some prescription drugs can be a matter of professional discretion, especially in the absence of strict guidelines from the manufacturer or the U.S. Food and Drug Administration. The heading Drug and

Food Interactions is not given for some drugs because no significant interactions have been noted for those drugs.

It is good practice not to keep outdated medicines on hand; which is why we suggest that you check the expiration date on all prescription bottles you have on hand and discard any medicines beyond the expiration date.

CHAPTER 15

Medicines for Infections

Antibiotics are a group of medicines that either destroy or inhibit the growth of bacteria causing an infection. In general, antibiotics have specific indications, that is, one type of antibiotic fights certain kinds of bacteria. Self-medication or transfer of medicine is not advisable even if symptoms appear to be familiar, because the underlying cause can be completely different.

The improper use of antibiotics may result in prolongation of the underlying infection and may even foster the development of additional bacteria to aggravate the existing illness. Another important point to remember about this class of drugs is that the disappearance of infectious symptoms may not mean the cure of the disease. In fact, stopping the medicine prematurely can lead to a recurrence of the illness or an even more severe form of infection. Therefore, it is necessary and even crucial to finish the total number of doses prescribed.

During prolonged antibiotic therapy (of weeks or months), bacteria resistance to the antibiotic may develop. Alternatively a condition known as superinfection may occur, in which a second infection erupts, superimposed upon the original infection for which the antibiotic was initially prescribed. This occurs because the organisms causing the second infection do not respond to the antibiotic already in the body. As the antibiotic disrupts the balanced growth of the bacterial populations in the body, organisms that existed in too small a number to produce disease now find the opportunity to grow and cause an infection. The prescriber should be contacted as soon as possible when the signs of an active infection recur, even if the prescribed antibiotic has been taken as directed.

Antibiotics should be taken at regular intervals throughout the day. When an antibiotic is prescribed for use three times a day, it is best to be taken every eight hours; if prescribed four times a day, take it every six hours. A young child may sleep ten to twelve hours a day, or a school-age child may spend eight hours in school, making such a schedule impractical. Depending on the circumstances, strict adherence to the ideal schedule may be unnecessary. Each case needs to be considered individually; the prescriber or the pharmacist should be consulted for a schedule best suited to the child as well as the disease under treatment. For a detailed discussion on the timing of dosages, see Chapter 1.

Commonly Prescribed Antibiotics

AMOXICILLIN

Trade Names: Amoxil, Amoxicillin, Augmentin, Larotid, Polymox, Sumox, Trimox, Utimox, Wymox.

Drug Class: Antibiotic.

Dosage Forms: Capsules, chewable tablets, suspension.

Available in Generic Form: Yes.

Why Used: For a variety of upper respiratory infections such as otitis media, sinusitis, epiglottitis, and pneumonia. Sometimes used for urinary tract infection as well.

How to Give:

- Usually prescribed to be taken three times a day, it is advisable to take it about thirty minutes before a full meal or an hour after. A light snack, such as an apple, a serving of ice cream, a cookie, or a granola bar, should not affect its absorption.
- When the capsule form is prescribed, it should be taken with a generous quantity (6 to 8 oz) of water.
- When the suspension is used, be sure to shake the bottle well before pouring out the medicine.

Unintended Effects:

- Occasionally loose stools occur in some children.
- Skin rash (itchy, red patches), but not common.

- Occasionally a yeast infection (superinfection) occurs in mouth or diaper area.

Contraindication: Previous allergy to ampicillin or other members of the penicillin family (e.g. cloxacillin, dicloxacillin, and penicillin).

Drug and Food Interaction: A full meal may reduce the absorption of amoxicillin.

Special Notes:

- Any uncomfortable reactions, such as loose stool or skin rash, should be discussed with the prescriber as soon as possible.
- It is important to finish the total amount prescribed; the prescriber should be notified of any reasons for stopping the drug.

Storage Instruction:

- Most liquid preparations should be kept refrigerated; however, leaving it at room temperature for one or two hours does not hurt the potency of the drug. Capsules should be kept at room temperature.
- Certain brands of the liquid preparation may not require refrigeration. If traveling with this drug is anticipated, consult the pharmacist for an alternative that does not need refrigeration.
- An expiration date should appear on the prescription bottle; if not, consult the pharmacist. Any unused portion should be discarded after the expiration date.

AMPICILLIN

Trade Names: Ampicillin, Amcill, Pfizerpen-A, Polycillin, Principen, SK-Ampicillin, Totacillin, Omnipen.

Drug Class: Antibiotic.

Dosage Forms: Capsule, suspension, injection.

Available in Generic Form: Yes.

Why Used: For a variety of upper respiratory infections such as otitis media, sinusitis, epiglottitis, and pneumonia. Sometimes used for urinary tract infection as well.

How to Give: Usually prescribed four times a day, it is advisable to take it about one hour before a full meal or two hours after. When the suspension is used, be sure to shake the bottle well before pouring out the medicine.

Unintended Effects:

- May induce diarrhea, especially in children under three. Consult prescriber if this occurs; however, diarrhea is usually self-limiting.
- Skin rash (itchy, red patches); more common in children with mononucleosis.
- Occasionally a yeast infection (superinfection) occurs in mouth and diaper areas.

Contraindication: Previous allergy to amoxicillin or other members of the penicillin family (e.g., cloxacillin, dicloxacillin, and penicillin).

Drug and Food Interaction: A full meal may reduce the absorption of ampicillin.

Special Note: Any uncomfortable reactions to this drug, such as loose stool or skin rash, should be discussed with the prescriber as soon as possible.

Storage Instructions:

- The liquid preparation should be kept refrigerated; however, leaving it at room temperature for one or two hours does not hurt the potency of the drug.
- If traveling with this drug is anticipated, consult the pharmacist for methods of storage.
- An expiration date should appear on the prescription bottle; if not, consult the pharmacist. Any unused portion should be discarded after the expiration date.

CEFACLOR

Trade Name: Ceclor.

Drug Class: Antibiotic.

Dosage Forms: Capsule, suspension.

Available in Generic Form: No.

Why Used: For a variety of infections, including otitis media, pneumonia, bone infection, skin infection, and urinary tract infection. Used as a substitute for penicillin or amoxicillin because of known allergy to either drug.

How to Give:

- Usually prescribed to be taken three to four times a day; absorption is not significantly affected by food.
- When the suspension is used, be sure to shake the bottle well before pouring out the medicine.
- It is important to finish the prescribed regimen. Prescriber should be notified of any reasons for stopping the drug.

Unintended Effects:

- Loose stools may occur occasionally.
- Skin rash (rare).
- Occasionally a yeast infection (superinfection) occurs in mouth or diaper area.

Contraindication: Previous allergy to this drug or cephalexin.

Special Notes:

- Any uncomfortable reactions to this drug, such as loose stools, skin rash, or yeast infection, should be discussed with the prescriber as soon as possible.
- Any child who suffered a previous allergy to a member of the penicillin family should take this drug with caution because of possible cross-sensitivity.

Storage Instructions:

- The liquid preparation should be refrigerated; however, leaving it at room temperature for one or two hours does not affect the potency of the drug. Capsules should be kept at room temperature.
- If traveling with the suspension is anticipated, consult the pharmacist for methods of storage.
- Expiration date should appear on the prescription bottle; if not, consult the pharmacist. Discard any unused portion of the drug after the expiration date.

CEPHALEXIN

Trade Name: Keflex.

Drug Class: Antibiotic.

Dosage Forms: Capsule, suspension.

Available in Generic Form: No.

Why Used: For a variety of infections, including otitis media, pneumonia, bone infection, skin infection, and urinary tract infection. Used as a substitute for penicillin or amoxicillin because of known allergy to either drug.

How to Give:

- Usually prescribed three to four times a day; absorption is not significantly affected by food.
- When the suspension is used, be sure to shake the bottle before pouring out the medicine.
- It is important to finish the prescribed regimen. Prescriber should be notified of any reasons for stopping the drug.

Unintended Effects:

- Loose stools may occur occasionally.
- Skin rash (rare).
- Occasionally a yeast infection (superinfection) occurs in mouth or diaper area.

Contraindication: Previous allergy to this drug or cefaclor.

Special Note: Any uncomfortable reactions to this drug, such as loose stools or skin rash, should be discussed with the prescriber as soon as possible.

Storage Instructions:

- The liquid preparation should be refrigerated; however, leaving it at room temperature for one or two hours does not affect the potency of the drug. Capsules should be kept at room temperature.
- If traveling with this drug is anticipated, consult the pharmacist for methods of storage.
- Expiration date should appear on the prescription bottle; if not, consult the pharmacist. Discard any unused portion after the expiration date.

CHLORAMPHENICOL

Trade Names: Chloramphenicol, Chloromycetin, Mychel.

Drug Class: Antibiotic.

Dosage Forms: Capsule, suspension, eyedrop and ointment, injection.

Available in Generic Form: Yes.

Why Used: For certain infections that are not easily treatable by other antibiotics, for example, periorbital cellulitis, bone infection in children under five years, meningitis, or epiglottitis.

How to Give:

- Well absorbed. Food does not significantly impede absorption of the drug.
- When the suspension is used, be sure to shake the bottle well before pouring out the medicine. If the capsule is prescribed, it can be opened and the contents mixed with a small serving of applesauce or ice cream for administration.
- It is important to finish the total amount prescribed; the prescriber should be notified of any reasons for stopping the drug.

Unintended Effects:

- Anemia can occur; periodic blood counts may be needed during prolonged therapy of four to six weeks.
- Occasional nausea, vomiting, and diarrhea.

Contraindication:

- Previous allergy to or a history of toxic effects from this drug.
- May aggravate existing blood or bone marrow disorder.

Special Note: Contact prescriber if tiredness, fever above 102° F, sore throat, bleeding, or unusual bruising develops during treatment with chloramphenicol.

Storage Instructions:

- Both suspension and capsules are kept at room temperature.
- Expiration date should appear on the bottle; if not, consult the pharmacist.
- Discard unused portion after expiration date.

COTRIMOXAZOLE OR TRIMETHOPRIM-SULFA

Trade Names: Bactrim, Bethaprim, Cotrim, Septra, Sulfatrim, SMZ-TMP

Drug Class: Antibiotic.

Dosage Forms: Tablet, suspension, injection.

Available in Generic Form: Yes.

Why Used: To treat a variety of infections, including otitis media, sinusitis, urinary tract infection, or certain types of diarrhea. Also used to prevent the occurrence of these infections.

How to Give:

- Usually prescribed twice a day; food does not significantly affect its absorption.
- Suspension should be shaken well before pouring out the medicine.
- It is advisable to take the drug with 4 to 6 ounces of fluid.

Unintended Effects:

- Occasionally causes upset stomach; food may alleviate the discomfort.
- Skin rash and hives, but not common.
- Anemia can occur; periodic blood count may be needed with long-term therapy of several weeks or months.

Contraindications:

- Anyone with known allergy to sulfa should not take this drug.
- Anyone with folate-deficiency anemia should not take this drug.

Special Notes:

- Contact prescriber if skin rash, fever, sore throat, mouth sores, unusual bleeding, or bruising occurs during prolonged therapy.
- Bacterial resistance may develop during prolonged therapy. Contact prescriber at the early signs of a recurrent infection (e.g., otitis media, urinary tract infection).

Storage Instructions:

- Both suspension and tablet are kept at room temperature.
- Expiration date should appear on the bottle, especially when long-term therapy is anticipated.

CLOXACILLIN

Trade Names: Cloxacillin, Cloxapen, Tegopen.

Drug Class: Antibiotic.

Dosage Forms: Capsule, suspension.

Available in Generic Form: Yes.

Why Used: Usually for skin infection, such as impetigo or boils.

How to Give:

- Should be taken one hour before or two hours after meals for optimal absorption.
- Even though the liquid preparation looks almost clear, it should be shaken before administration.
- If the capsule is used, it can be opened and the contents mixed with a small serving of applesauce or ice cream for administration.

Unintended Effects:

- Occasionally causes upset stomach.
- Skin rash, but this is not a common reaction.

Drug and Food Interaction: A full meal may reduce the absorption of cloxacillin.

Contraindications:

- Previous allergy to this drug or other members of the penicillin family.
- Anyone with known allergy to a cephalosporin antibiotic (such as cefaclor or cephalexin) should take this drug with caution because of possible cross-sensitivity.

Special Notes:

- Any uncomfortable reactions to this drug, such as loose stool or skin rash, should be discussed with the prescriber as soon as possible.
- It is important to finish the total amount prescribed; prescriber should be notified of any reasons for stopping the drug.

Storage Instructions:

- The liquid preparation should be refrigerated, but leaving it at room temperature for one or two hours does not affect the potency of the drug. Capsules should be stored at room temperature.
- Expiration date should appear on the prescription bottle; if not, consult the pharmacist. Discard unused portion after expiration date.
- For long-term therapy of four to six weeks and if traveling is anticipated, the capsule can be used instead of the suspension for convenience.

DICLOXACILLIN

Trade Names: Dicloxacillin, Dycill, Dynapen, Pathocil, Veracillin.

Drug Class: Antibiotic.

Dosage Forms: Capsule, suspension.

Available in Generic Form: Yes.

Why Used: Usually for skin infection, such as impetigo or boils, as well as for bone infection.

How to Give:

- Should be taken one hour before or two hours after meals for optimal absorption.
- The suspension is a thick liquid; it should be shaken thoroughly before pouring out the medicine.
- If the capsule is used, it can be opened and the contents mixed with a small serving of applesauce or ice cream for administration.

Unintended Effects:

- Occasionally causes upset stomach.
- Skin rash, but this is not a common reaction.

Drug and Food Interaction: A full meal may reduce the absorption of dicloxacillin.

Contraindications:

- Previous allergy to this drug or other members of the penicillin family.
- Anyone with known allergy to a cephalosporin antibiotic (such as cefaclor or cephalexin) should take this drug with caution because of possible cross-sensitivity.

Special Notes:

- Any uncomfortable reactions to this drug, such as loose stool or skin rash, should be discussed with the prescriber as soon as possible.
- It is important to finish the total amount prescribed; prescriber should be notified of any reasons for stopping the drug.

Storage Instructions:

- The liquid preparation should be refrigerated, but leaving it at room temperature for one or two hours does not affect the potency of the drug. Capsules should be stored at room temperature.
- Expiration date should appear on the prescription bottle; if not consult the pharmacist. Discard unused portion after expiration date.
- For long-term therapy of four to six weeks and if traveling is anticipated, the capsule can be used instead of the suspension for convenience.

ERYTHROMYCIN

Trade Names: Bristamycin, Ery-Ped, Ery-Tab, E.E.S., E Mycin, Erythrocin, Erythromycin, Ilosone, Ilotycin, Pediamycin, Pfizer E, Robinmycin, SK-Erythromycin, Wyamycin E.

Drug Class: Antibiotic.

Dosage Forms: Capsule, enteric-coated, chewable and film-coated tablet, suspension, injection.

Available in Generic Form: Yes.

Why Used: For a variety of respiratory infections such as otitis media, sinusitis, pneumonia, and skin infections. Also used as an alternative to penicillin in patients with penicillin allergy.

How to Give:

- Coated tablets of erythromycin should not be cut or crushed, since this will expose the core of the tablet and inactivate it in stomach acid.
- If the suspension is used, be sure to shake the bottle before pouring out the medicine.

Unintended Effects:

- Occasionally causes upset stomach.
- Skin rash occurs rarely.

Drug and Food Interactions:

- Certain brands of erythromycin can be taken with food without affecting absorption. Consult pharmacist on brand selection.
- If your child is already taking theophylline, be sure to let the prescriber know when erythromycin is added because of possible interaction between these two drugs.

Contraindication: Previous allergy to this drug.

Special Notes: Contact prescriber if severe abdominal pain, yellow discoloration of skin or eyes, darkened urine, or unusual tiredness occurs.

Storage Instructions:

- Suspension and tablets can be kept at room temperature. Refrigeration enhances the flavor of the liquid, making it more palatable for children.
- Expiration date should appear on the bottle; if not, consult pharmacist.

GRISEOFULVIN

Trade Names: Fulvicin P/G, Fulvicin-U/F, Grifulvin V.

Drug Class: Antifungal.

Dosage Forms: Tablet (micro and macro crystal), suspension.

Available in Generic Form: Yes.

Why Used: For a variety of fungal skin infections involving the hair and nails.

How to Give:

- Usually prescribed to be taken once a day.
- Dose should be taken with a fatty meal for optimal absorption (dinner rather than breakfast).
- It is important to finish the prescribed regimen.

Unintended Effects:

- Occasionally causes nausea, vomiting, and stomachache.
- Skin rash, but not common.
- May cause sunburn in individuals who are excessively exposed to sunlight or sun lamp while on therapy (photosensitivity).

Drug and Food Interaction: Fatty food enhances the absorption of griseofulvin.

Contraindication: Previous allergy to this drug.

Special Notes:

- Anyone with known allergy to penicillin should take griseofulvin with caution because of possible cross-sensitivity between the two drugs. Advise the prescriber if griseofulvin is prescribed and your child is allergic to penicillin.
- Contact prescriber if fever, sore throat, or skin rash occurs.
- Griseofulvin tablet comes in two types: one contains the large (macro) crystals and the other, small (micro) crystals. The latter is much better absorbed and may be less costly in the long run because the dose can be reduced by half, for instance, a 250 mg small crystal tablet is approximately equal in strength to a 500 mg large crystal tablet.

Storage Instructions:

- Both tablets and suspension are kept at room temperature.
- Expiration date should appear on the bottle, especially when long-term therapy is anticipated.

MEBENDAZOLE

Trade Name: Vermox.

Drug Class: Anthelmintic (antiworm).

Dosage Form: Chewable tablet.

Available in Generic Form: No.

Why Used: For treatment of hookworm, pinworm, whipworm, or mixed worm infestation.

How to Give:

- Tablet may be chewed, crushed, or swallowed.
- Can be given at any time of day.

Unintended Effects:

- Occasional diarrhea and abdominal pain.
- Fever (rare).

Contraindication: Previous allergy to this drug.

Special Notes:

- Be sure to follow the prescribed regimen for complete elimination of worms.
- The symptoms of worm infestation are general and varied. Consult your health care provider for a confirmed diagnosis rather than attempting to medicate your child.

Storage Instructions: Tablets are kept at room temperature.

Age Limitation: Not recommended for children under two years.

METRONIDAZOLE

Trade Names: Flagyl, Metronidazole, Metryl, Protostat, Satric.

Drug Class: Antibiotic.

Dosage Forms: Tablet, injection.

Available in Generic Form: Yes.

Why Used: For treatment of specific types of parasitic infection, for instance, trichomoniasis, amebiasis of the intestine or other organs.

How to Give: May be taken with food to alleviate the nauseating effect.

Unintended Effects:

- Nausea, vomiting, and upset stomach are common, and the medicine also leaves a metallic taste in mouth.
- May darken color of urine.
- May cause headache, dizziness, or numbness of extremities (rare).

Drug and Food Interaction: Your child should avoid alcohol-containing beverages while on this therapy, because alcohol interacts with the drug and results in some uncomfortable reactions. Alcohol may be present in some medicinal formulations such as cough drops. Consult the pharmacist for information on alcohol-containing medicines.

Contraindication: Previous allergy to this drug.

Special Note: Be sure to follow the prescribed regimen for complete eradication of infection.

Storage Instructions:

- Tablets are kept at room temperature.
- Consult pharmacist for expiration date of the drug if none appears on package.

NITROFURANTOIN

Trade Names: Furadantin, Furalan, Furan, Furante, Furatoin, Macrodantin.

Drug Class: Antibiotic.

Dosage Forms: Capsule (macro crystal and regular), tablet, suspension.

Available in Generic Form: Yes.

Why Used: Primarily for treatment or prevention of urinary tract infection.

How to Give:

- Should be taken with food to minimize discomfort to the stomach as well as for maximal absorption.
- When the suspension is prescribed, shake the bottle well before pouring out the medicine.

Unintended Effects:

- Commonly causes upset stomach or abdominal pain.
- Pneumonialike allergic reaction in lungs (rare).

Contraindications:

- Previous allergy to this drug.
- Severe kidney disease.

Special Notes:

- Contact prescriber if fever, chills, cough, difficult breathing, skin rash, or numbness of extremities occurs.
- Available in two types: one contains the large crystals (macro) and the other contains the regular size crystals. The former is better absorbed and less likely to cause upset stomach but it is more costly than the regular size crystals.

Storage Instructions:

- Tablet, capsule, and suspension are kept at room temperature.
- Expiration date should appear on the prescription bottle if long-term therapy lasting weeks to months is anticipated.

NYSTATIN

Trade Names: Nilstat, Nystatin, Mycostatin.

Drug Class: Antifungal.

Dosage Forms: Tablet (oral and vaginal), suspension, cream, ointment, and powder.

Available in Generic Form: Yes.

Why Used: For fungal or yeast infection of mouth—such as thrush—vagina, or skin.

How to Give:

- Usually prescribed to be taken three or four times a day, at any time of the day before or after meals, since the effect of the drug is achieved by contact with the infected body part, not by absorption into the body.
- The vaginal tablet is sometimes prescribed as a lozenge for oral thrush. It offers the advantage of slow dissolution in the mouth and thus provides a longer period of contact.
- When the suspension is used, for optimal result each dose should be retained in the mouth for several minutes before spitting out or swallowing. If your child is too young to do this, an alternative is to use a cotton swab and paint the medicine on the infected surface. Then discard the used swab and use a clean swab for a second application, if needed. Be sure to shake the bottle before pouring out the medicine.
- When prescribed as a powder, cream, and ointment for topical application,

make sure the infected area is clean prior to application, especially when it is used for diaper rash. Consult your health care provider in the case of chronic and persistent diaper rash.

Unintended Effects: Occasionally causes upset stomach.

Contraindication: Previous allergy to this drug.

Special Notes:

- Fungal infection can be stubborn and difficult to cure. Thus it is important to follow the regimen prescribed for your child and to complete the entire course of therapy. Continue treatment for forty-eight hours after there is no more evidence of the rash or thrush unless instructed otherwise.
- The Mycostatin brand of the oral suspension has a high sugar content of 50 percent dextrose. If sugar is undesirable, consult prescriber or pharmacist for a different brand.

Storage Instructions:

- Both solid and liquid preparations are kept at room temperature.
- Expiration date should appear on the bottle; if not, consult pharmacist.

PENICILLIN

Trade Names: Beepan-VK, Betapen-BK, Ledercillin VK, Pen-Vee K, Penapar VK, Pentids, Pfizerpen VK, Robicillin VK, SK-Penicillin VK.

Drug Class: Antibiotic.

Dosage Forms: Tablet, suspension, injection.

Available in Generic Form: Yes.

Why Used: For a variety of upper respiratory infections, such as strep throat, ear infection, and pneumonia.

How to Give:

- Should be taken one hour before or two hours after a full meal.
- Be sure to shake the bottle well before pouring out the medicine.

Unintended Effects:

- Infrequent sensitivity reaction may occur in the form of skin rash or, in severe cases, tightness of chest, wheezing, swelling of the mouth and throat. Notify prescriber immediately if any of these occurs.
- Occasionally causes nausea, vomiting, and upset stomach.

Drug and Food Interaction: A full meal may reduce the absorption of penicillin.

Contraindications:

- Previous allergy to this drug or other members of the penicillin family (e.g., ampicillin, amoxicillin, cloxacillin, dicloxacillin).
- Anyone with known allergy to a cephalosporin antibiotic, such as cefaclor or cephalexin, should take penicillin with caution because of possible cross-sensitivity.

Storage Instructions:

- The liquid preparation requires refrigeration, whereas the tablet is kept at room temperature.
- Expiration date should appear on the bottle; if not, consult pharmacist. Discard any unused portion after the expiration date.

RIFAMPIN

Trade Names: Rifadin, Rimactane.

Drug Class: Antibiotic.

Dosage Form: Capsule.

Available in Generic Form: Yes.

Why Used: In combination with other antibiotics, to treat tuberculosis or as prevention against meningitis.

How to Give: Usually prescribed to be taken once or twice a day; may be taken before or after meals.

Unintended Effects:

- Occasionally causes upset stomach.
- Skin rash and hives, but not common.

Contraindication: Previous allergy to this drug.

Special Notes:

- This drug imparts an orange-red or brown color to body secretions such as urine, feces, saliva, sweat, or tears. Do not be alarmed, because this is not harmful to the body.
- Available commercially in capsule form only; the liquid form requires special preparation by a pharmacist.

Storage Instructions:

- Capsule is kept at room temperature.
- If a liquid preparation is specially made, refrigeration is required.
- Expiration date should appear on the bottle; if not, consult pharmacist.

SULFISOXAZOLE

Trade Names: Gantrisin, Sulfisoxazole, SK-Soxazole.

Drug Class: Antibiotic.

Dosage Forms: Tablet, suspension, eyedrop, ointment.

Available in Generic Form: Yes.

Why Used: In combination with another antibiotic for otitis media or urinary tract infection.

How to Give:

- Food has little effect on its absorption; thus it may be taken before or after meals.
- Offer your child plenty of fluids to drink when taking this medicine.
- When the suspension is prescribed, shake the bottle well before pouring out the medicine.

Unintended Effects:

- Occasionally causes nausea, vomiting, and upset stomach.
- Skin rash or a more generalized form of skin inflammation.

Contraindication: Previous allergy to this drug.

Special Notes: Make note of any unusual reactions (e.g., skin rash) to this medicine, since sulfisoxazole is related to another drug that is found in combination with still another drug that goes by a different name. For example, Bactrim or Septra is a sulfa-containing drug that should be avoided if your child has a known allergy to sulfa.

Storage Instructions:

- Both liquid and tablets are kept at room temperature.
- Expiration date should appear on bottle; if not, consult pharmacist. This is especially important if long-term therapy is anticipated, such as in the case of prevention against recurrent otitis media or urinary tract infection.

TETRACYCLINE

Trade Names: Achromycin V, Cyclopar, Panmycin, Robitet, SK-Tetracycline, Sumycin, Tetrachel, Tetracyn, Tetracycline.

Drug Class: Antibiotic.

Dosage Forms: Capsule, suspension, ointment, injection.

Available in Generic Form: Yes.

Why Used: For a variety of infections, including acne, sinus and lung infection.

How to Give:

- For treatment of acne it is usually prescribed to be taken once or twice a day for extended periods.
- For other infections it is mostly prescribed to be taken three or four times a day for a limited course, such as ten days.
- It is best taken one hour before or two hours after a meal.

Unintended Effects:

- Commonly causes nausea, vomiting, and upset stomach.
- Treatment with tetracycline may lead to overgrowth of fungal infection (superinfection) in mouth and vagina in some susceptible teenagers.
- May cause sunburn in individuals who are excessively exposed to sunlight or sun lamp while on therapy (photosensitivity).

Drug and Food Interactions: Do not give your child dairy products (milk, cheese) antacids (Maalox, Pepto-Bismol, Riopan), or iron tablets to take with tetracycline because they bind with the drug and impair its absorption.

Contraindications:

- Children under eight years should not take tetracycline since it can cause staining of the permanent teeth.
- Previous allergy to this drug.

Storage Instructions:

- Capsules and suspension are kept at room temperature.
- Expiration date should appear on the bottle; if not, consult pharmacist This is especially important when long-term therapy is anticipated, as in the case of treatment of acne.

Age Limitation: Not recommended for children under eight years.

TRIMETHOPRIM-SULFA. SEE COTRIMOXAZOLE OR
TRIMETHOPRIM-SULFA.

CHAPTER 16

Medicines for Seizure and Behavioral Control

This chapter describes the medicines that are commonly prescribed for control of seizures and behavioral disorders. Some of these drugs fall into the category of controlled substances, as defined by the Federal Controlled Substances Act, because of their high abuse potential. It is good practice to take special precaution in the storage of such medicines in case your child wants to or is tempted to share them with friends.

Commonly Prescribed Medicines

CARBAMAZEPINE

Trade Name: Tegretol.

Drug Class: Anticonvulsant.

Dosage Forms: Tablet (chewable and regular).

Available in Generic Form: No.

Why Used: For convulsive disorder, either partial seizure or the generalized tonic-clonic type, characterized by stiff jerking movements of the body or the extremities.

How to Give:

- Chewable tablet should be chewed before swallowing.
- Take with food for better absorption.

Unintended Effects:

- Drowsiness, especially when therapy first begins; dizziness and unsteady gait.
- May affect bone marrow production of white blood cells. Periodic blood counts are usually done.
- Consult the prescriber should the following symptoms develop: skin rash, excessive fatigue, loss of appetite, or disorientation.

Drug and Food Interactions: Carbamazepine may interact with other anticonvulsant drugs such as phenytoin, phenobarbital, valproic acid, and clonazepam. Hence, drug levels should be checked periodically to monitor therapy and modify dosage accordingly.

Contraindications:

- Existing liver disease.
- Previous allergy to this drug.
- Severe blood disorders.

Special Notes:

- Control of seizures is dependent on taking the drug regularly as prescribed. Full effect of seizure control or reduction may not be apparent for one to two weeks after beginning drug therapy.
- It is advisable for the child to wear a protective helmet if seizures occur frequently despite therapy.
- School personnel should be informed of the child's history of seizures. If the drug is prescribed to be taken three times a day, the school nurse should be notified to administer the dose or to remind the child to do so.

Storage Instructions:

- Keep at room temperature.
- Expiration date of the drug should appear on the bottle; otherwise consult the pharmacist.

CLONAZEPAM

Trade Name: Clonopin.

Drug Class: Anticonvulsant.

Dosage Form: Tablet.

Available in Generic Form: No.

Why Used: For seizure control (petit mal seizures).

How to Give:

- May be taken before or after meals.
- If prescribed to be taken twice a day, give one dose in the morning and one dose at bedtime.

Unintended Effects:

- Irritability and drowsiness, which may subside with continued therapy.
- Occasionally, behavioral changes; your child may become aggressive or agitated, for example.
- Skin rash (rare).
- Stomach discomfort occasionally occurs. It can be alleviated by giving your child a snack.

Drug and Food Interactions:

- The drowsiness effect of this drug may be enhanced by the concurrent intake of medicines with sedative property, such as certain cold remedies.
- The addition of other anticonvulsant medicines, such as carbamazepine and valproic acid, to clonazepam therapy may affect seizure control in the child.

Contraindications:

- Existing liver disease.
- Previous allergy to this drug or to other members of the benzodiazepine family (e.g., Valium, Librium).

Special Notes:

- Effectiveness may diminish as the child develops a tolerance for this drug. Early signs of this are increased occurrence of seizure. At this time the dose may need to be raised or alternative treatment considered.
- Consult the prescriber if excessive drowsiness and fatigue becomes evident, especially when other drugs, such as phenobarbital or cold remedies, are taken at the same time.
- Also notify the prescriber if seizure frequency has increased noticeably after the addition of other anticonvulsant drugs, such as carbamazepine or valproic acid.
- It is advisable for the child to wear a protective helmet if seizures occur frequently despite therapy.

Storage Instructions:

- Tablets are kept at room temperature.
- Consult the pharmacist for expiration date of the drug.

CODEINE

Trade Name: None for codeine as a single drug.

Drug Class: Narcotic analgesic, antitussive.

Dosage Forms: Elixir, tablet, injection.

Available in Generic Form: Yes.

Why Used: To decrease pain or cough.

How to Give:

- Take with food to alleviate discomfort to the stomach.
- Take only as needed rather than regularly unless instructed otherwise by your health care provider.

Unintended Effects:

- Drowsiness, lightheadedness, and sedation are common.
- May cause upset stomach and constipation (both effects are common).
- Skin rash (rare).

Drug and Food Interactions:

- The drowsiness effect is enhanced by the concurrent use of other agents with sedative properties like cold remedies.
- Intensifies the intoxicating effect of alcohol or alcohol-containing medicines.

Contraindication: Previous allergy to this drug or other members of the opiate family (e.g., morphine, meperidine).

Special Notes:

- This medicine may be habit forming if used for prolonged periods (weeks).
- Tolerance to the sedative effect of this drug varies, so the same dose may have different effects on different children.
- Encourage fluid intake with each dose to reduce the constipating effect.

Storage Instructions:

- Both the elixir and the tablets are kept at room temperature.
- Codeine is a controlled substance; be sure to keep this in a safe place.
- Consult the pharmacist for expiration date of the drug.

DEXTROAMPHETAMINE

Trade Name: Dexedrine.

Drug Class: Stimulant.

Dosage Forms: Capsule (sustained-release), tablet.

Available in Generic Form: No.

Why Used: For nyperactivity or attention deficit disorder (ADD). While it seems puzzling that a stimulant is used to treat hyperactivity, to date there is enough clinical evidence to demonstrate that some children with hyperactivity can benefit from stimulant therapy.

How to Give: When prescribed to be taken once a day, the single daily dose should be taken after breakfast or as early in the day as possible. If a twice-a-day schedule is prescribed, the second dose should be taken before 4 P.M. each day to avoid insomnia at night.

Unintended Effects:

- Suppresses appetite, usually during initial therapy.
- Nervousness, headache, and irritability. May cause insomnia, especially during initial therapy.
- Quite commonly, withdrawal depression when the medicine is stopped may result in tearfulness or crying for no apparent reason.
- Infrequently, increases heart rate, although some children are more susceptible to this effect than others.

Drug and Food Interactions: Vitamin C enhances the excretion of dextroamphetamine if taken concurrently in a large dose of 1 gm of vitamin C or more. Antacids containing sodium bicarbonate, such as Alka-Seltzer, reduce its excretion, resulting in prolonged action.

Contraindication: Previous allergy to this drug.

Special Notes:

- ADD is a clinical diagnosis that requires careful investigation by a health professional rather than a casual labeling on the basis of the child's activity. This is usually done by psychological testing, attention span studies, and other clinical tests.
- Both the family and the schoolteacher have to work together with the health care provider to determine if the child may benefit from drug therapy.

- While there is no evidence of addiction among those who receive the drug for ADD, tolerance may develop, requiring dose adjustment.
- The child's growth and weight should be monitored carefully in case the appetite-suppressant effect may impede growth.
- If the sustained-release capsule cannot be swallowed whole, the contents may be emptied for administration, but they should not be crushed or chewed.

Storage Instructions:

- This is a controlled substance because of its abuse potential; be sure to keep it in a safe place.
- Keep at room temperature.
- Usually a small quantity is prescribed each time, such as a one- to two-month supply; it is unlikely that the drug will deteriorate before it is consumed.

ETHOSUXIMIDE

Trade Name: Zarontin.

Drug Class: Anticonvulsant.

Dosage Forms: Capsule, syrup.

Available in Generic Form: No.

Why Used: For seizure control (petit mal seizure).

How to Give: May be taken before or after a meal, depending on the stomach's reaction.

Unintended Effects:

- Drowsiness, dizziness, or irritability are common.
- Upset stomach occurs commonly.

Contraindication: Previous allergy to this drug.

Special Notes:

- Should be taken as directed; sporadic intake may jeopardize seizure control.
- The school nurse should be notified to either administer the drug or to remind the child to do so if one of the doses is to be taken in school.
- Consult prescriber if frequency of seizures seems to increase after initiation of therapy.

- Capsule cannot be taken apart; if your child has difficulty swallowing it, the liquid preparation can be prescribed instead.
- It is advisable for the child to wear a protective helmet if seizures occur frequently despite therapy.

Storage Instructions:

- Both capsule and liquid, a syrup, are kept at room temperature.
- Since control of seizures usually requires long-term treatment, the expiration date of the drug should appear on the bottle.

HYDROXYZINE

Trade Names: Atarax, Vistaril.

Drug Class: Antihistamine.

Dosage Forms: Capsule, coated tablet, syrup, suspension, injection.

Available in Generic Form: No.

Why Used: For anxiety or to lessen allergic reaction.

How to Give:

- Usually to be taken as needed rather than on a regular basis. It is best taken at bedtime for its sedative and antiitching effects.
- When the drug is used as a sedative prior to a clinical procedure such as dental work, it is best to be taken thirty minutes to one hour prior to the appointment.
- If the suspension is prescribed, be sure to shake the bottle well before pouring out the medicine.
- Do not attempt to crush the coated tablet if your child cannot swallow the tablet whole. Consult the prescriber for alternative dosage forms.

Unintended Effect: Drowsiness is common.

Drug and Food Interactions: Enhances the drowsiness effect of other drugs with sedative properties when taken at the same time.

Contraindication: Use with caution in children with uncontrollable seizures.

Special Notes:

- Useful in treatment of skin inflammations, to decrease constant scratching, which can result in infection.

- If your child is already taking other drugs, be sure to notify the prescriber when hydroxyzine is added in case of possible interactions.

Storage Instructions:

- The capsule, tablet, syrup, and suspension are all kept at room temperature.
- Hydroxyzine may be taken as needed rather than regularly; hence a supply of the drug may last some time. Consult the pharmacist for the expiration date.

IMIPRAMINE

Trade Names: Imavate, Imipramine HCL, Janimine, Presamine, SK-Pramine, Tofranil.

Drug Class: Antidepressant.

Dosage Forms: Coated tablet, capsule, injection.

Available in Generic Forms: Yes.

Why Used: Although it is classified as an antidepressant, its most common use in children is for treatment of bed-wetting (enuresis) in an age group that is usually toilet-trained (school age or older).

How to Give:

- When prescribed once a day, give the dose at bedtime.
- Do not attempt to crush the coated tablet if your child cannot swallow it whole. Consult the prescriber for methods of administration or alternative forms of therapy.

Unintended Effects:

- Drowsiness is common.
- Dry mouth and constipation are also quite common.

Drug and Food Interactions:

- Vitamin C enhances the excretion of this drug when taken together in a large dose such as 1 gram of vitamin C or more.
- Antacids containing sodium bicarbonate, such as Alka-Seltzer, reduce its excretion, resulting in prolonged effect of the drug.

Contraindication: This drug should be used with caution in a child with known seizure disorder or heart disease.

Special Notes:

- Bed-wetting is a traumatic experience for a child; hence it should be treated with understanding and careful consideration. Sometimes it could be due to a functional disorder of the urinary tract that renders bladder control difficult or impossible. If that has been ruled out and bed-wetting continues, then a trial of therapy with imipramine can be helpful.

- Despite the drug class it belongs to, imipramine has no stimulant effect.

Storage Instructions:

- Keep at room temperature.
- Since this drug may be taken on a trial basis to begin with, it is advisable to know the expiration date at the time drug therapy begins.

Age Limitation: Not indicated for children under six years.

METHYLPHENIDATE

Trade Name: Ritalin.

Drug Class: Stimulant.

Dosage Form: Tablet.

Available in Generic Form: No.

Why Used: For treatment of hyperactivity or attention deficit disorder (ADD). While it seems puzzling that a stimulant is used to treat hyperactivity, to date there is enough clinical evidence to demonstrate that some children with hyperactivity can benefit from stimulant therapy.

How to Give: The tablet is usually prescribed to be taken twice a day. The first dose should be taken after breakfast or as early in the day as possible and the second dose before 4 P.M. each day to avoid insomnia at night.

Unintended Effects:

- May suppress appetite during initial therapy, but this effect is less prominent than with dextroamphetamine.
- Nervousness, headache, and irritability are common; may occasionally cause insomnia.
- Withdrawal depression when the medicine is stopped may result in tearfulness or crying for no apparent reason.
- Possible slowing of growth rate.

Contraindications:

- Should be taken with caution in the presence of cardiac disease.
- Previous allergy to this drug.

Special Notes:

- Attention deficit disorder is a clinical diagnosis that requires a careful investigation rather than a casual labeling on the basis of the child's activity level. This is usually done by psychological testing, attention span studies, and other clinical tests. Both the family and the schoolteacher have to work together with the health care provider to determine if the child may benefit from drug therapy.
- While there is no evidence of addiction among those who receive the drug for ADD, tolerance may develop, requiring dose adjustment.
- The child's growth and weight should be monitored carefully.

Storage Instructions:

- This is a controlled substance because of its abuse potential; be sure to keep it in a safe place.
- Keep at room temperature.
- Since usually a small quantity is prescribed each time, such as a one- to two-months supply, it is unlikely that the drug will deteriorate before it is consumed.

PEMOLINE

Trade Name: Cylert.

Drug Class: Stimulant.

Dosage Form: Tablet (chewable and regular).

Available in Generic Form: No.

Why Used: For treatment of hyperactivity or attention deficit disorder (ADD). While it seems puzzling that a stimulant is used to treat hyperactivity, to date there is enough clinical evidence to demonstrate that a select group of ADD patients can benefit from stimulant therapy.

How to Give: Usually prescribed to be taken once a day, to be taken as early in the day as possible to avoid insomnia at night.

Unintended Effects:

- Usually suppresses appetite during initial therapy.
- Nervousness, headache, and irritability may occur, especially in the first week of therapy.
- Growth rate may slow.

Contraindication: Previous allergy to this drug.

Special Notes:

- ADD is a clinical diagnosis that requires careful investigation by a health professional rather than a casual labeling on the basis of the child's activity level. This is usually done by psychological testing, attention span studies, and other clinical tests. Both the family and the schoolteacher have to work together with the health care provider to determine if the child may benefit from drug therapy.
- While there is no evidence of addiction among those who receive the drug for ADD, tolerance may develop and require dose adjustment.
- The child's growth and weight should be carefully monitored.

Storage Instructions:

- This is a controlled substance; be sure to keep it in a safe place.
- Keep at room temperature.
- Pemoline is not as tightly controlled as dextroamphetamine or methylphenidate because of its lesser abuse potential; therefore more than a one- to two-months supply may be prescribed each time. Be sure to ask the pharmacist for the expiration date of the drug dispensed.

PHENOBARBITAL

Trade Names: Barbital, Henotal, Luminal, Phenobarbital, SK-Phenobarbital.

Drug Class: Anticonvulsant, sedative.

Dosage Forms: Elixir, tablet, injection.

Available in Generic Form: Yes.

Why Used: For seizure control.

How to Give:

- The total daily dose may be taken once a day at bedtime; however, if divided doses are prescribed, do not change the schedule without consulting the prescriber.
- The elixir contains alcohol; taking it with food alleviates discomfort to the stomach.

Unintended Effects:

- Sedation and drowsiness are common.
- Occasionally after taking phenobarbital, a child may become excitable and restless rather than sedated.

Drug and Food Interaction: Medicines with sedative properties such as over-the-counter antihistamines enhance the drowsiness effect of phenobarbital.

Contraindications:

- Severe obstructive lung disease.
- Previous allergy to this drug or other members of the barbiturate family.

Special Notes:

- This drug is not addicting to a child with seizure disorder; thus for optimal result it should be taken as directed rather than sporadically or whenever a seizure occurs.
- When given orally, phenobarbital does not stop the seizure instantly. The drug level in the body has to be built up gradually and maintained to prevent seizures from occurring. Do not discontinue taking the medicine abruptly if the child is on treatment for an extended period of time, such as months to years.
- Consult the prescriber if the child appears to be excessively sleepy and walks unsteadily.
- Prescriber should be aware of other drugs the child is taking concurrently with phenobarbital, especially other anticonvulsant drugs, because of possible interactions.
- The elixir contains both sugar and alcohol.

Storage Instructions:

- This is a controlled substance; be sure to keep it in a safe place.
- Both tablet and elixir are kept at room temperature.
- Since treatment of seizures requires long-term therapy, it is helpful to be aware of the expiration date of the drug.

PHENYTOIN

Trade Names: Dilantin, Di-Phenylan, Di-Phen, Ditan, Phenytoin Sodium.

Drug Class: Anticonvulsant.

Dosage Forms: Capsule, chewable tablet, suspension, injection.

Available in Generic Form: Yes.

Why Used: For seizure control.

How to Give:

- When the suspension is prescribed, be sure to shake the bottle well before pouring out the medicine.
- Chewable tablet should be chewed or crushed before swallowing.
- The total daily dose can be taken once a day at bedtime; however, if divided doses are prescribed, do not change the schedule without consulting the prescriber.

Unintended Effects:

- Drowsiness is common during initial therapy; this should diminish in time.
- May occasionally cause upset stomach.
- Skin rash or skin inflammation occurs occasionally. Excessive growth of facial hair or acne has also occurred in some children.
- Overgrowth of gum. Some children are more prone to this than others. Daily dental hygiene (brushing and flossing) is important in reducing these changes and chances for infection. Frequent dental checkups are also advisable. Such care is especially important in the child whose permanent teeth have developed.

Drug and Food Interactions: The addition of folic acid or phenobarbital to phenytoin therapy may affect its anticonvulsant activity.

Contraindication: Previous allergy to this drug.

Special Notes:

- Notify the prescriber if the child appears to be excessively sedated and sleepy or walks unsteadily, especially when other anticonvulsant drugs such as phenobarbital are added to phenytoin therapy.
- Periodic blood counts and drug levels in blood are used to monitor therapy.
- If any of the following symptoms occur, contact the prescriber as soon as possible: dark urine, yellow tint to the skin, loss of appetite, stomach pain, sore throat, bruises on the skin, nosebleed.
- Phenytoin produced by different companies may create different blood levels in the body. Consult the prescriber on the choice of a preferred brand. Once determined, stay with it for the duration of therapy.
- The full effect of seizure control may not be apparent for one to two weeks.

Storage Instructions:

- The tablet, capsule, and suspension are all kept at room temperature.
- Since the treatment of seizure requires long-term therapy, it is advisable to have the expiration date of the drug on the bottle.

PRIMIDONE

Trade Names: Mysoline, Primidone.

Drug Class: Anticonvulsant.

Dosage Forms: Tablet, suspension.

Available in Generic Form: Yes.

Why Used: For seizure control.

How to Give:

- Taking the drug with food alleviates discomfort to the stomach.
- If the suspension is prescribed, be sure to shake the bottle before pouring out the medicine.

Unintended Effects:

- Drowsiness is common during initial therapy. It should subside over time.
- May cause upset stomach, which may subside after the medicine has been given for some time.

Contraindication: Previous allergy to this drug or phenobarbital.

Special Notes:

- Periodic checks of drug levels in blood are used to monitor therapy.
- Consult the prescriber if your child appears excessively sedated and sleepy or walks unsteadily.
- Should be taken regularly as directed rather than sporadically or whenever seizure occurs. The full effect of seizure control may not be apparent for two to three weeks. For optimal result the drug level has to be built up gradually and maintained to prevent the occurrence of seizures.

Storage Instructions:

- Both tablet and suspension are kept at room temperature.
- Treatment of seizure requires long-term therapy; it is advisable to have expiration date on the bottle.

VALPROIC ACID

Trade Name: Depakene.

Drug Class: Anticonvulsant.

Dosage Forms: Capsule, syrup.

Available in Generic Form: No.

Why Used: For seizure control.

How to Give: Taking it with food alleviates discomfort to the stomach. Capsules cannot be taken apart; if your child has difficulty swallowing them, the liquid preparation can be prescribed instead.

Unintended Effects:

- Drowsiness is common, especially when the child is on multiple-drug therapy for seizure control.
- Stomach discomfort is common; may be alleviated with food.

Drug and Food Interactions:

- The addition of other anticonvulsant drugs such as phenobarbital, phenytoin, or clonazepam may affect the anticonvulsant activity of valproic acid.
- This medicine may interfere with urine tests for ketones in diabetics.

Contraindication: Previous allergy to this drug.

Special Notes:

- Periodic blood counts and drug levels in blood are used to monitor therapy.
- Contact the prescriber if any of the following symptoms develop: bruises on the skin, loss of appetite, stomach pain, excessive sedation.
- Prescriber should be aware of drugs that are taken at the same time for seizure control because of possible interactions.

Storage Instructions:

- Both capsule and syrup are kept at room temperature.
- Control of seizure requires long-term treatment; it is advisable to know the expiration date of the drug.

CHAPTER 17

Medicines for the Heart and Lungs

Medicines in this chapter are commonly prescribed for the treatment of heart and lung disorders. These are to be differentiated from those in Chapter 9 in two ways:

1. These drugs require a prescription.
2. These drugs are more potent and require the continual monitoring of a health care provider.

Commonly Prescribed Cardiac and Respiratory Medicines

ALBUTEROL

Trade Names: Proventil, Ventolin.

Drug Class: Bronchodilator.

Dosage Forms: Tablet, oral inhaler.

Available in Generic Form: Yes.

Why Used: For asthma or other airway obstructive disease.

How to Give:

- Print instructions are available in the package insert, which should accompany the oral inhaler when dispensed by a pharmacist. Be sure to obtain such instructions for use or to have a demonstration from your health care provider before your child begins using it.

- Usually prescribed for inhalation every four to six hours or at the onset of an asthmatic attack. More frequent use than the prescribed regimen increases the incidence and severity of unintended effects.

Unintended Effects:

- Dizziness and headache are common during initial therapy.
- May occasionally increase heart rate; some children are more susceptible than others to this effect.

Contraindications:

- Use with caution in a child with irregular heart rhythm or heart disease.
- Previous allergy to this drug.

Special Notes:

- For optimal result your child should learn to use the inhaler properly. Consult the pharmacist for detailed instructions.
- School personnel should be aware of your child's need for a bronchodilator to avoid misunderstanding when it is used occasionally in school.
- When the oral inhaler is used at the onset of an asthmatic attack, relief of breathing difficulty usually occurs within fifteen to thirty minutes.

Storage Instructions:

- Kept in original container at room temperature.
- Expiration date should appear on the bottle.

CHLOROTHIAZIDE

Trade Names: Chlorothiazide, Diachlor, Diuril, SK-Chlorothiazide.

Drug Class: Diuretic.

Dosage Forms: Tablet, suspension, injection.

Available in Generic Form: Yes.

Why Used: To lessen the work load for the heart and the kidneys by eliminating excess salt and fluid from the body.

How to Give:

- Usually prescribed to be taken once or twice a day. The first dose should be taken in the morning and the second dose before 4 P.M. so it does not interfere with the child's sleep due to increased urination. If the child is not yet toilet trained, frequent changing of diapers may be necessary.

- If the suspension is prescribed, shake the bottle well before pouring out the medicine.

Unintended Effects: May result in electrolyte imbalance in the body, which may cause excessive fatigue, lack of energy, severe constipation, and muscle weakness. These are the usual symptoms of low amounts of potassium in the body.

Contraindications: Previous allergy to this drug or other members of the family, for example, sulfa drug.

Special Notes:

- A diuretic gets rid of excessive salt (sodium) in the body. In the process of doing so, it also eliminates potassium. To replenish the lost potassium, the following foods are recommended unless the child is on a restricted diet: orange or citrus juice, tomatoes, prunes, raisins, bananas, peanut butter, all-bran cereal, meat.
- The diuretic effect of this drug is quite immediate, usually taking 1 to 2 hours.
- Contact the prescriber if the child shows excessive fatigue, lack of energy, severe constipation, or muscle weakness. This is especially important if the child is also on digitalis (digoxin) therapy.
- If the child has vomiting or diarrhea or any other dehydrating illness, contact the prescriber.

Storage Instructions:

- Both the tablet and suspension are kept at room temperature.
- It is advisable to have the expiration date on the bottle.

CROMOLYN

Trade Names: Aarane, Intal, Nasalcrom.

Drug Class: Bronchospasmolytic.

Dosage Forms: Capsule (for inhalation only), nasal solution.

Available in Generic Form: Yes.

Why Used: To prevent constriction of bronchioles in the lungs, which can lead to asthmatic attack and certain kinds of allergies.

How to Give: The capsule is for inhalation use with a spinhaler only. It is not for oral use.

Unintended Effects:

- Throat irritation due to the powder from inside the capsule. Dry mouth and possibly chest tightness may occur occasionally.
- Irritation of the nose (a burning or stinging sensation or even sneezing) when the nasal solution is used.
- May occasionally cause upset stomach.

Contraindication: Previous allergy to this drug.

Special Notes:

- Cromolyn is to be used regularly to prevent an asthmatic attack. However, it should not be used during the attack, since it has no direct effect on the bronchioles and the irritation effect may even worsen the attack.
- If asthma is brought about by exercise, then the drug should be given thirty minutes prior to exercise.
- In some special situations cromolyn may be prescribed for oral use, but its primary use is for inhalation by mouth.
- It is important for the child to know how to use the spinhaler in order to benefit from the drug; otherwise it may have no effect. Printed instructions should accompany the inhaler when dispensed by a pharmacist. Be sure to ask for such instructions or a demonstration from your health care provider before your child begins using it.
- Throat irritation can be minimized by a few swallows of water following each inhalation.

Storage Instructions:

- Keep at room temperature in original container.
- It is advisable to know the expiration date of the drug due to its infrequent use by some children.
- Clean spinhaler following use as directed on the label of the container.

DIGOXIN

Trade Names: Digoxin, Lanoxin, Lanoxicaps.

Drug Class: Heart stimulant.

Dosage Forms: Elixir, tablet, capsule, injection.

Available in Generic Form: Yes.

Why Used: For heart failure or rhythm regulation.

How to Give:

- Can be taken with food except by young infants, who may regurgitate after feeding, making it hard to determine how much of a dose needs to be replaced.
- Take one dose in the morning if prescribed for daily use or once in the morning and once at bedtime if prescribed to be taken twice daily.

Unintended Effects: It slows down heart rate.

Drug and Food Interactions:

- Food high in bran fiber may reduce the absorption of digoxin in the intestine.
- If your child takes a diuretic at the same time as digoxin, the potassium level in the body may need to be checked periodically. This is done by a blood sample taken by your health care provider.
- If your child takes a potassium supplement at the same time as digoxin, the potassium level in the body may also need to be checked periodically, because too high a potassium level may impede the cardiac activity of digoxin.

Contraindication: Previous allergy to this drug or other members of the digitalis family, such as digitoxin.

Special Notes:

- Too slow a heart rate can be undesirable in a child with heart failure; some prescribers suggest that the parent measure the pulse rate prior to each dose. Check for recommendations from your prescriber.
- Consult the prescriber if your child shows lack of appetite, vomiting, diarrhea, or change in activity level.
- Some prescribers check the drug level in the body periodically to monitor therapy, especially if the child is taking other drugs concurrently, such as a diuretic.
- Potency of digoxin tablets can vary with different manufacturers. Consult the prescriber on the choice of a brand. Once determined, it is advisable to stay with the same brand for the duration of therapy.
- If an excess dosage is inadvertently administered or accidentally taken, contact your Poison Control Center immediately.

Storage Instructions:

- Both tablet and elixir are kept at room temperature.
- This is a potent medicine. Be sure to keep it out of reach of all children.
- Because of the small dose a child takes, a bottle may last a long time. It is advisable to have the expiration date of the drug on the bottle.

FUROSEMIDE

Trade Names: Furosemide, Lasix, SK-Furosemide.

Drug Class: Diuretic.

Dosage Forms: Elixir, tablet, injection.

Available in Generic Form: Yes.

Why Used: To lessen the work load for the heart and the kidneys by eliminating excess salt and fluid from the body.

How to Give:

- When prescribed to be taken once a day, give the dose in the morning. When prescribed twice a day, give the second dose before 4 P.M. to avoid interfering with the child's sleep due to increased urination. If your child is not yet toilet trained, more frequent changing of diapers may be necessary.
- May be taken before or after a meal.

Unintended Effects: May cause electrolyte imbalance in the body; usually manifested by excessive fatigue, lack of energy, severe constipation, and muscle weakness. These are indicative of a low potassium level in the body. Contact the prescriber for advice.

Drug and Food Interactions: When your child takes furosemide and digoxin at the same time, the potassium level in the body may need to be checked periodically.

Contraindication: Previous allergy to this drug.

Special Notes:

- A diuretic gets rid of excessive salt (sodium) and fluid from the body. In the process of doing so it also eliminates potassium. To replenish the lost potassium, the following food items are recommended unless the child is on a restricted diet: orange or citrus juice, tomatoes, prunes, raisins, bananas, all-bran cereal, peanut butter, meat.
- The diuretic effect of this drug is immediate, usually one to two hours.

- If the child appears excessively tired, lacking in energy, and has severe constipation and muscle weakness, contact the prescriber. These may be signs of a low potassium level in the body.

Storage Instructions: The liquid form should be kept refrigerated. After opening the bottle, it is good for sixty days unless you are advised otherwise by the pharmacist. The tablet is kept at room temperature.

METAPROTERENOL

Trade Names: Alupent, Metaprel.

Drug Class: Bronchodilator.

Dosage Forms: Tablet, syrup, oral inhaler, solution for inhalation.

Available in Generic Form: Yes.

Why Used: For asthma or other airway obstructive diseases.

How to Give:

- The aerosolized inhaler is usually prescribed for use every four to six hours or at the onset of an asthmatic attack. More frequent use of the inhaler than prescribed increases the incidence and severity of unintended effects. For best results the child should learn to use the inhaler properly. Consult the pharmacist for detailed information.
- The tablet and syrup are usually prescribed for use as needed rather than regularly. The oral dose should not be given more often than every four to six hours unless you are instructed otherwise by the prescriber.

Unintended Effects:

- Headache and nervousness are common during initial therapy and become more pronounced with increased use.
- Increased heart rate and flushing of the face occur occasionally, and the incidence goes up with more frequent use of inhaler.

Contraindications:

- Use with caution in a child with severe heart disease.
- Previous allergy to this drug.

Special Notes:

- It is important for the child to know how to use the inhaler in order to benefit from the drug; otherwise it may have no apparent effect and may even lead to increased use and unintended effects. Printed instructions should accompany the inhaler when dispensed by a pharmacist. Be sure to ask for such instructions or to have a demonstration by your health care provider before your child begins using it.

- School personnel should be aware of your child's need for a bronchodilator to avoid misunderstanding, since the child may require an occasional dose in school.
- When the oral inhaler is used, relief of breathing difficulty usually comes within fifteen to thirty minutes.

Storage Instructions:

- The inhaler in its original container, the tablet and the syrup are all kept at room temperature.
- It is advisable to know the expiration date, since a supply of the drug may last a long time, especially if it is used only as needed.

PROPRANOLOL

Trade Name: Inderal.

Drug Class: Heart rhythm regulator.

Dosage Forms: Tablet, injection.

Available in Generic Form: No.

Why Used: To treat irregular heartbeat.

How to Give: May be taken before or after a meal.

Unintended Effects:

- Slows down the heart rate, which may aggravate existing congestive heart failure.
- Fatigue and lightheadedness (especially when standing up quickly from a sitting position) are common.

Drug and Food Interactions:

- When propranolol and digoxin are taken at the same time, heart rate may become unusually slow; it is important to monitor the pulse periodically.
- May decrease the effect of some bronchodilators, such as metaproterenol, terbutaline, possibly albuterol and theophylline.

Contraindications:

- Use with caution in asthmatics, diabetics, and children with heart failure.
- Previous allergy to this drug.

Special Notes:

- Propranolol masks the symptoms of low blood sugar; monitor urine sugar more closely if your diabetic child also needs propranolol.
- The smallest dose that can be given in tablet form is 2.5 mg, which is one-quarter of a 10 mg tablet. If a smaller dose than this is needed, it requires special preparation by a pharmacist.
- Some prescribers may want you to omit a dose if the child's heart rate goes below a certain range; it is advisable to discuss this with the prescriber. If you must take your child's pulse rate while she or he is on this medicine, ask the health care provider to demonstrate the correct way.

Storage Instructions:

- The tablet is kept at room temperature.
- Expiration date should be on the bottle in case it is stopped for a while and resumed because of changes in heart condition.

SPIRONOLACTONE

Trade Names: Alatone, Aldactone, Spironolactone.

Drug Class: Diuretic.

Dosage Form: Tablet.

Available in Generic Form: Yes.

Why Used: To lessen the work load for the heart and the kidneys by eliminating excess sodium and fluid from the body without severely depleting the body of potassium. Also used for certain special liver conditions.

How to Give: May be taken before or after a meal.

Unintended Effects:

- May cause electrolyte imbalance in the body, which is usually manifested by numbness of the extremities, fatigue, muscle weakness, and slow heart rate.
- Drowsiness and headache occur occasionally.
- Irregular menses occurs occasionally.
- Skin rash occurs rarely.

Drug and Food Interactions:

- Despite its diuretic action, spironolactone does not deplete the body of potassium; hence, potassium supplement is usually not needed even when your child is on prolonged therapy. Sometimes it is even used with one of the other diuretics to conserve potassium in the body.
- Digoxin level may need to be monitored more closely with the addition of this drug because of its effect on potassium balance in the body.

Contraindications:

- Should not be used with any preexisting condition of excess body potassium, such as kidney failure.
- Previous allergy to this drug.

Special Notes:

- The smallest dose available is 6.25 mg, which is one-quarter of a regular 25 mg tablet. If a smaller dose is needed, it requires special preparation by a pharmacist.
- The tablet has a minty flavor; it should be kept away from children who may mistakenly take it for candy.

Storage Instructions:

- The tablet is kept at room temperature.
- The expiration date should appear on the bottle, since the clinical condition may change before the supply of tablets is consumed.

TERBUTALINE

Trade Names: Brethine, Bricanyl.

Drug Class: Bronchodilator.

Dosage Forms: Tablet, injection.

Available in Generic Form: Yes.

Why Used: To prevent and treat asthma by relaxing bronchiole muscles.

How to Give:

- May be taken before or after a meal.
- It may be prescribed on an as-needed basis. Allow two to three hours between doses if it is used only during an asthmatic attack.

Unintended Effects:

- Nervousness and headache are common during initial therapy.
- Increases heart rate; the effect is prominent in susceptible children.

Contraindications:

- Previous allergy to this drug.
- Severe heart disorder or irregular heart rhythm.

Special Notes:

- If asthma is brought about by exercise, a dose should be taken thirty minutes prior to exercise. When the oral tablet is taken prior to an asthmatic attack, the bronchodilation effect usually occurs within an hour.
- School personnel should be aware of the child's need for a bronchodilator to avoid misunderstanding if the child needs to take the medicine in school.
- Do not exceed the recommended dosage; excessive use may lead to increased incidence and severity of unintended effects.

Storage Instructions:

- Keep at room temperature.
- It is advisable to know the expiration date, since a supply may last a long time if it is used only occasionally.

THEOPHYLLINE

Trade Names: Aerolate, Bronkodyl, Elixophyllin, Elixicon, Slo-bid, Slo-Phyllin, Somophyllin-T, Theolair, Theophylline, Theo-Dur, Theo-bid, Theophyl.

Drug Class: Bronchodilator.

Dosage Forms: Capsule (regular and sustained-release), tablet (regular and sustained-release), elixir, syrup, suspension, injection, enema.

Available in Generic Form: Yes.

Why Used: A bronchodilator which relaxes the bronchiole muscle to make breathing easier.

How to Give:

- If the drug is prescribed for regular use, it should be taken as directed. For some children it is prescribed for use only during or to prevent an asthmatic attack.
- Taking theophylline with food alleviates discomfort to the stomach.
- If the suspension is prescribed, shake the bottle well before pouring out the medicine.
- If the tablet is a sustained-release preparation, it should not be crushed;

  if the instruction is for taking one-half of the tablet, consult the pharmacist
  on how to divide it evenly.
- If a sustained-release capsule is prescribed, the capsule can be opened
  and the inside granules swallowed whole rather than chewed.

Unintended Effects:

- Nervousness, headache, and irritability are common during initial therapy;
  however, if these symptoms become excessive, consult the prescriber for
  dosage adjustment.
- Increased heart rate; may be more prominent in some children.

Drug and Food Interactions:

- Concurrent treatment with erythromycin may enhance the effect of
  theophylline.
- Taking the medicine immediately after a full, fatty meal may alter the
  absorption pattern of the sustained-release tablet or capsule. It is advisable
  to give the medicine one to two hours after a fatty meal if your child
  takes one of these dosage forms.
- When phenobarbital is taken in addition to theophylline, it may alter the
  bronchodilation activity of theophylline.

Contraindication: Previous allergy to this drug.

Special Notes:

- The diversity of dosage forms is intended to suit individual needs. If your
  child experiences unintended effects with a certain type of theophylline,
  consult the prescriber or the pharmacist for alternatives.
- During an asthmatic attack a child may not be able to swallow a dose of
  the medicine for relief; a retention enema is available for such an occasion.
  The suppository preparation, on the other hand, has fallen into disuse
  because of unreliable absorption.
- The sustained-release formulation is most appropriate for daily therapy
  when the child's asthma is controlled. Some health care providers may
  prescribe a short-acting brand of theophylline for occasional emergency
  use. Become well versed with the instructions for administration before
  stress and anxiety set in during an emergency.
- It is important to take theophylline as directed because of its potential
  serious unintended effects.
- For optimal result, drug concentration in the body should be within a
  certain range; for this reason blood tests are warranted periodically.
- Contact the prescriber in the event of excessive vomiting, stomach pain,
  restlessness, and irritability.
- Some theophylline preparations contain sugar and alcohol, which may
  cause an upset stomach. Take with plenty of fluids to minimize the
  discomfort.

- Avoid colored liquid preparations if your child is allergic to food dye.
- Be sure to inform the prescriber if any new drugs are added to the child's regimen, because of possible interactions.
- Bronchodilation effect should be apparent within an hour after taking the short-acting tablet; with the sustained-release preparation, it may take one to two hours.

Storage Instructions:

- Keep at room temperature.
- It is advisable to know the expiration date of the drug in case it is used only occasionally.

Common Equivalents

Household	Metric	Apothecaries'
volume		
1 teaspoon (tsp)	5 cubic centimeters (cc) or 5 milliliters (ml)	1 fluidram (fl dr)
1 tablespoon (tbsp) or 3 tsp	15 cc or 15 ml	4 fl dr
1 cup	180 cc	6 fluid ounces (fl oz)
1 glass	240 cc	8 fl oz
weight		
	1 kilogram (kg)	2.2 pounds (lb)
	60 milligrams (mg)	1 grain (gr)
	30 mg	½ gr

These are approximate equivalents of weights and volumes among metric, apothecaries', and household systems that are useful in giving medications. It is important to remember that they are approximate and not exact equivalents. Some loss of accuracy occurs whenever one system of measure is converted to another.

Metric Equivalents

500 milligrams (mg) = 0.5 gram or ½ gram (gm)

1000 mg   = 1 gm

Conversion of Human Temperatures from Fahrenheit to Centigrade

Fahrenheit (degrees)	Centigrade (degrees)
93.2	34.0
95.0	35.0
96.8	36.0
98.6	37.0
100.4	38.0
102.2	39.0
104.0	40.0
105.8	41.0
107.6	42.0
109.4	43.0

From Malasanos, L., et al. *Health Assessment,* 2nd ed., 1981, p. 139.

How to Use a Bulb Syringe to Suction an Infant's Nose

Young infants and small children are unable to blow their noses to rid them of mucus. Thus mucus tends to accumulate in the nasal passages when they have a cold. This mucus becomes dry and crusted and will impede breathing. Since infants are nose breathers, it becomes important to clear the nasal passages, especially before feeding.

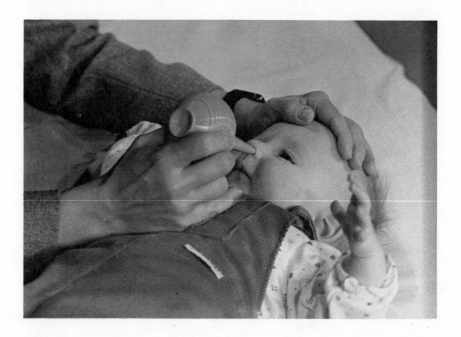

Saline nosedrops are used to soften the dry mucus in an infant's nose and facilitate its removal. A bulb syringe is then used to remove the mucus gently. This is done by deflating the bulb, gently inserting it into the nostrils, and gradually releasing pressure from the bulb so that the suctioning action pulls the mucus into the bulb. After clearing one nostril, expel all the mucus removed from the nose into a tissue and repeat the procedure with the other nostril in the same manner. The child may cry and usually does not like this, so you may need to mummy-restrain the child as described in Chapter 4 to control the arms and legs. Use your free hand to stabilize the child's head. Always make sure the child cannot squirm or fall off the surface wherever you are doing this procedure.

After the nostrils are cleaned, you can complete the feeding. Following the feeding, wash the bulb syringe well in hot soapy water. Rinse the syringe well and dry it. Use only one syringe per child to avoid transferring the germs carried on the syringe.

Home First-Aid Supplies

Thermometer
Scissors
Tweezers
Sterile gauze (2″ × 2″ and 4″ × 4″)
Gauze roller bandage
Elastic roller bandage
Paper tape
Triangular bandage
Ice bag
Hot water bottle
Child medicine spoon and/or syringe
Aspirin
Acetaminophen
Syrup of ipecac
Activated charcoal
Rubbing alcohol
Calamine lotion
Strips of cloth ⎫
Flat pieces of wood ⎭ For splints

Glossary

acute Sudden and short, usually referring to the outbreak and course of a disease, as opposed to *chronic*.

ADD Attention deficit disorder, commonly known as hyperactivity.

adsorbent A chemical that binds to the surface of other substances, including bacteria and toxins; this is how it works to inactivate the harmful substances.

allergy Increased sensitivity to certain foreign substances to which the body is exposed. The result can be manifested in a variety of symptoms involving different body organs, the most common being tearing, hives, skin rashes, and itchiness. These can progress to swollen tongue and eyelids, shortness of breath (due to obstruction of the airway by the swollen tongue), and shock.

analgesic Pain killer.

Antabuse reaction Describes reactions following the combined ingestion of the drug Antabuse and alcohol. In the presence of alcohol in the body, Antabuse produces flushing, headache, breathing difficulty, nausea, increased heart rate, weakness, confusion, and fainting.

antibiotic A class of drugs that destroys germs or stops their growth.

anticonvulsant A drug used to control seizures (convulsions).

antifungal A kind of chemical that destroys yeasts specifically or stops their growth.

anthelmintic A drug used to treat worm infection.

antitussive A drug used to stop coughing.

bronchodilator A drug used to expand the breathing vessels in the lungs; commonly used to treat conditions such as asthma and chronic lung obstruction.

bronchospasmolytic A drug used to relieve or prevent spasm of the breathing vessels in the lungs.

cellulitis Skin infection.

chronic Slow and continuous, usually referring to the course of a disease. A condition that lasts a long time is described as chronic.

congenital Condition present at birth.

contraindication Reason for which a medicine should not be given.

corticosteroids A class of drugs used to treat inflammatory conditions.

cough Sudden and forceful expulsion of air or irritating substance from the throat. When only air comes up, it is a dry or unproductive cough, usually due to irritation in the throat. When sputum is coughed up, it is a productive cough.

cross-sensitivity When two drugs have similar chemical structures or origin and a child has an allergy to one of them, it is possible that he or she may also be allergic to the other.

decongestants Medicines that reduce nasal congestion or discharge due to increased secretion.

diuretic A drug used to rid the body of excessive fluid, thus lessening the workload on the heart.

eczema Inflammatory skin disease.

edema Swelling due to accumulation of fluid in the body tissue.

electrolytes Substances that are necessary for certain cellular functions in the body. Examples are potassium and sodium.

elixir Alcohol-containing liquid vehicle for medicinal use.

enteric coating Special surface coating to protect the contents of a tablet from being destroyed by stomach acid; in this way, the chemical structure of the drug will remain intact to carry out its pharmacological action.

enuresis Bed-wetting; urinating in sleep after being toilet-trained.

epiglottitis Inflammation of the larynx.

expectorant Medicine that loosens secretion in the lungs to make it easier to be expelled.

expiration date The date after which the potency or quality of a drug may deteriorate.

fatigue Tiredness, lack of energy.

hyperactivity Increased activity; generally referring to a condition observed in children characterized by restlessness, short attention span, impulsivity, and learning disabilities. This is also known as attention deficit disorder (ADD) or minimal brain dysfunction (MBD).

hyperextension Stretching of a part of the body, such as the neck or an arm, beyond 180°.

hypersecretory Increased secretion of fluid.

hypersensitivity Increased sensitivity; equivalent to allergy.

inflammatory response A reaction to a foreign substance, including medicines, characterized by redness, swelling, pain, and heat.

inspiratory Breathing in.

K cal Kilocalorie, a measurement unit of calories.

keratolytic A substance that causes disintegration of skin epidermis.

macro or **micro crystal** *Macro* is big, *micro* is small; both refer to the size of the crystal, the basic structure of a chemical.

otitis externa Inflammation of the ear canal.

otitis interna or **labyrinthitis** Inflammation inside the ear.

otitis media Middle ear infection.

otoscope Instrument used to look inside the ear.

osteomyelitis Bone infection.

pallor Pale color.

paradoxical Opposite result.

periorbital cellulitis   Skin infection around the eye resulting in pronounced swelling of the skin surrounding the eye.

pH   Degree of neutrality of the chemical nature of a solution; a solution with a pH of 7 is neutral, above 7 is alkaline, below 7 is acidic.

pharmacological   Related to the actions of a drug on the body.

photophobia   Intolerance to light, especially strong light.

photosensitive   Allergic to sunlight, usually due to the action of certain drugs.

physiological   Dealing with the function of the human body.

pneumonia   Lung infection.

projectile vomiting   Vigorous vomiting to such a degree that the vomitus is forcefully expelled from the stomach rather than just drooled.

prophylaxis   Treatment to prevent the occurrence of an infection, such as taking rifampin after exposure to meningitis.

psychogenic   Originating from the mind or emotions.

psychological   Relating to what goes on in the mind rather than in the body.

psychosocial   Originating from or affecting both the mind and the social environment.

rebound congestion   Continual and frequent use of nasal decongestants can lead to overstimulation and constriction of the blood vessels in the nasal cavities; as a natural response, the blood vessels will bounce back by dilating as soon as the drug effect subsides. As a result, this becomes a cyclical condition and the congestion will never improve.

self-limiting   Describes a condition that is not worsening in severity and symptoms.

sensitizing reaction   Allergic reaction.

solubility   Ability of being dissolved or going into solution.

superinfection   Synonymous with secondary infection; an infection following a previous infection, either with the same or a different organism.

suppository   A form of medication, elongated in shape, that contains medicine in a waxy coating. This is used for insertion into the rectum, vagina, or urethra.

suspension   A liquid preparation in which the ingredients are not completely dissolved. To mix the suspended articles with the liquid, the bottle needs to be shaken well immediately before use.

sustained release   A special formulation designed to release gradually the active ingredients from the core of a tablet inside the intestine.

vasoconstriction   Narrowing of blood vessels.

Selected Readings

Breast-feeding

La Leche League International. *The Womanly Art of Breast Feeding.* Franklin Park, Ill.: La Leche League International, 1982.

Everything you want to know about breast-feeding in a detailed but easy-to-read book.

Eiger, Marvin S., M.D., and Olds, Sally Wendkos. *The Complete Book of Breast-feeding.* New York: Workman Publishing Co., 1972.

An easy, readable book that covers many of the common questions mothers have about breast-feeding.

Child Rearing

Behrstock, Barry, M.D. *The Parents' When-Not-To-Worry Book.* New York: Harper and Row, 1981.

Examines and refutes many of the commonly accepted ideas and child-care practices. Presents the rationale and truth about these ideas in easily understood language.

Brazelton, T. Berry, M.D. *Doctor and Child.* New York: Delacorte Press/Seymour Lawrence, 1976.

Written by a pediatrician who has sensitive insight into the family's most common problems during early childhood. He gives practical, easy to follow advice.

Fraiberg, Selma. *The Magic Years.* New York: Charles Scribner, 1959.

A discussion of a child's mind from birth to six years that is a fascinating and readable approach to child development.

Ginott, Haim G., M.D. *Between Parent and Child.* New York: MacMillan Publishing Co., 1965.

A classic that still applies to today's youth. Explores discipline, jealousy, and anxiety in children and how parents can approach the situation and make the relationship between parents and children more rewarding.

Ginott, Haim G., M.D. *Between Parent and Teenager.* New York: MacMillan Publishing Co., 1969.

A sequel to the previous book written to deal with the problems facing the family with an adolescent.

Salk, Lee, Ph.D. *What Every Child Would Like His Parents to Know.* New York: David McKay Company, 1972.

Factual, straightforward advice on everything from working mothers and toilet training to dealing with a child in trouble. Stresses how to approach the situation while protecting the child's emotional health.

Discipline

Gibson, Janice T., Ed.D. *Discipline Is Not A Dirty Word—A Positive Learning Approach.* Lexington, Mass.: The Lewis Publishing Co., 1983.

Emphasizes the positives of discipline and focuses on the parent as the role model. Deals with the problems of not only the younger child but the adolescent as well.

Child Development

Brazelton, T. Berry, M.D. *Infants and Mothers.* New York: Dell Publishing Co., 1981.

Parents receive insights into their own baby's unique personality. Active, quiet, and average baby characteristics are discussed for the first year of life.

Caplan, Frank and Teresa. *The First Twelve Months of Life.* New York: Perigee Books, The Putnam Publishing Group, 1973.

Gives a month-by-month description of how an infant develops physically, socially, and psychologically. Excellent illustrations.

Caplan, Frank and Teresa. *The Second Twelve Months of Life.* New York: Perigee Books, The Putnam Publishing Group, 1979.

A sequel to the previous book, also with a month-by-month presentation.

Caplan, Frank and Teresa. *The Early Childhood Years—The 2-6-Year-Old.* New York: Perigee Books, The Putnam Publishing Group, 1983.

A sequel to the previous two books, with the child's development presented in several-month spans.

White, Burton L. *The First Three Years of Life.* New York: Avon Books, 1975.

Informative development book on the first thirty-six months of a child's life. Discusses the needs of both the child and her or his parent.

Emergency and Medical Care Information

American Red Cross. *Standard First Aid and Personal Safety.* Garden City, N.Y.: Doubleday and Co., 1979.

A complete book of first aid that covers both the child and the adult.

Boston Children's Medical Center and Feinbloom, Richard, M.D. *Child Health Encyclopedia—The Complete Guide For Parents.* New York: A Delta Special/ Seymour Lawrence Book, 1978.

Covers common illness, injuries, and problems seen in children. Gives helpful medical advice for home care and tells you when you should seek professional assistance. It also includes a section on recommended car safety restraints for children.

Green, Martin I. *A Sigh of Relief: the first-aid handbook for Childhood Emergencies.* Toronto: Bantam Books, 1977.

A quick source of first-aid information presented in outline form. It also has large illustrations for easy reference.

Samuels, Mike and Nancy. *The Well Baby Book.* New York: Summit Books, 1979.

Methods for promoting the health of babies, beginning before birth, are discussed. Home care for minor illness, with alternatives to medicine treatment, is presented.

The Diagram Group. *Child's Body.* New York: Paddington Press, 1977.

This practical, readable book outlines development, child care, and health care. Many illustrations contribute to its clarity.

Medications

American Pharmaceutical Association. *Handbook of Nonprescription Drugs.* 7th ed. Washington, D.C.: American Pharmaceutical Association, 1982.

American Society of Hospital Pharmacists. *Consumer Drug Digest.* New York: Facts on File, 1982.

Boston Women's Health Book Collective. *The New Our Bodies, Our Selves.* 2d ed. New York: Simon and Schuster, 1985.

Bressler, R.; Bogdonoff, M.; and Subak-Sharpe, G., eds. *The Physicians' Drug Manual: Prescription and Nonprescription Drugs.* Garden City, New York: Doubleday and Company Inc., 1981.

Long, J. *The Essential Guide to Prescription Drugs.* New York: Harper and Row, 1985.

Physicians' Desk Reference for Nonprescription Drugs. 6th ed. Oradell, N.J.: Medical Economics Co., 1985.

Zimmerman, D. *The Essential Guide to Nonprescription Drugs.* New York: Harper and Row, 1983.

Parenthood

Brazelton, T. Berry, M.D. *On Becoming a Family.* New York: Dell Publishing Co., 1981.

This noted pediatrician discusses the development of attachment between baby and parents.

Kappelman Murray, M.D., and Acherman, Paul, Ph.D. *Parents After Thirty.* New York: Rawson, Wade Publishers, 1980.

Assists in answering questions of this age group when they are deciding to have children. Deals with impact of parenting on careers and lifestyles.

Salk, Lee, Ph.D. *Preparing for Parenthood.* New York: David McKay Company, 1974.

Focuses on conceiving a child in an emotional atmosphere where he or she is wanted. Salk provides information about deciding whether to become parents and gives psychological preparation for the father and mother through pregnancy, labor, and postpartum. Bonding between parents and child is also discussed.

Sullivan, S. Adams. *The Father's Almanac.* Garden City, N.Y.: Doubleday and Co., 1980.

The father's involvement in birth and child care is encouraged from pregnancy onward. Learning and play activities with children are described.

Special Considerations

The Unit at the Fayerweather Street School, Eric Rofes, editor. *The Kid's Book of Divorce.* New York: Vintage, 1982.

Twenty students whose parents experienced divorce or who thought their parents were divorcing came together to discuss their feelings and the impact it was having on their lives. They wrote this book for other children, under the supervision of the editor.

Index

Aarane, 275
abdominal pain
  laxatives and, 126–135
  minerals and, 107, 108
  vitamins and, 97
absorbents, 207–209
Absorbotear, 171
absorption, 3–5
  effectiveness and, 5
  of inhaled drugs, 4
  of injected drugs, 4
  of orally administered drugs, 3–4
  in rectum, 5
  of topically applied drugs, 4–5
accidental ingestion, 18
  of antihistamines, 148
  prevention of, 20, 28
  of sedatives, 148
acetaminophen, 83, 88, 89–90
  breast-feeding and, 11
  for fever, 87, 89
  for inflammation, 89
  for menstrual discomfort, 229–230
  for pain, 88–89
  in pregnancy, 11
  after vaccinations, 75
Achromycin, 199
Achromycin V, 256
acid indigestion, 136
Acnaveen Cleansing Bar, 197
acne, 196
  benzoyl peroxide for, 197
  retinoic acid for, 98, 196
  salicylic acid for, 197
  sulfur for, 198
  tetracycline for, 196, 257

Acne Aid, 198
Acnederm, 198
Acne-Dome, 198
Acno, 197
Acnomead, 198
Acnomel, 198
Acnotex, 197
activated charcoal, 138–139
active immunity, 72–73
Acutrim, 215
ADD (attention deficit disorder)
  dextroamphetamine for, 262
  methylphenidate for, 266
  pemoline for, 267
  vitamin C and, 103
addiction
  to laxatives, 125, 127–135
  to opiates, 123, 153, 261, 263
administration of medicines
  to adolescents, 29–30
  capsules, 33–36, 38
  for ears, 55–57
  to eyes, 48–55
  for hair, 60–65
  to infants, 27, 37–40
  liquid medicines, 31–33, 37–38
  by mouth, 31–42
  by nose, 57–60
  to preschoolers, 28–29
  by rectum, 43–48
  to school-age children, 29, 41–42
  for skin, 60–65
  tablets, 33–36
  to toddlers, 27–28, 40
  vaginal, 65–67

adolescents (twelve- to eighteen-year-olds)
    administering medicine to, 29–30
    alcohol and, 42
    constipation in, 125–126
    eardrops for, 57
    eye medicines for, 55
    illicit drugs and, 42
    nosedrops for, 59, 61
    skin disorders of, 195–196
    suppositories for, 48
    vaginal medicines for, 65–67
    vomiting by, 118
Advil, 92, 232
Aerolate, 283
Afko-Lube, 127
Afrin, 156
Aftate, 205
Agoral Plain, 131
Akne Drying, 197
A/K/Rinse, 176
Alatone, 281
albuterol, 273–274
alcohol, 87, 189
    adolescents and, 42
    breast-feeding and, 11
    fetus affected by, 10
    medicines interacting with, 30, 42, 148,
        153, 252, 261
Alconefrin 12, 157
Alconefrin 25, 157
Aldactone, 281
Alermine, 150
alkaline borate, 172
Alka-Seltzer, 90, 230
Alka-2, 136
Alkets, 135
Aller-Chlor, 150
Allerest, 151, 158
Allerest Eye Drops, 173
Allerest Nasal, 157
allergies, 60
    eyes affected by, 173
    immunizations and, 71
    to medicines, 9–10, 32
    to milk, 120
    side effects confused with, 9–10
Alophen Pills, 132
Alphalin, 97
Alphamul, 127
AlternaGEL, 136
Alucap, 136
Aludrox, 135
aluminum hydroxide, 136
Aluminum Hydroxide Gel, 136
Alupent, 279
Alu-Tab, 135
alveoli, 142
Amcill, 241

amebiasis, 251
amenorrhea, 224–226
American Academy of Pediatrics, 35, 96
American Medical Association, 32
American Pediatric Association, 96
aminobenzoic acid, 210–211
Amitone, 136
Ammens Medicated Powder, 208
ammonium chloride, 233
Amogel PG, 123
amoxicillin, 240–241, 255
Amoxil, 240
Amphojel, 135
ampicillin, 9, 241–242
A-M-T, 135
Anacin, 90, 230
analgesics, 83–93, 282–283
anaphylaxis, 9
anemia
    aplastic, 78
    folate-deficiency, 245, 246
    iron and, 110
    vitamins and, 102, 105
aniline dyes, 211
anorexia nervosa, 215
Anorexin, 215
Antabuse, 42
antacids, 111, 126, 135–138
anthelmintics, 251
antibiotics
    for acne, 196, 199–200
    for colds, 145
    diarrhea and, 120
    immunizations and, 71
    for infections, 239–257
    therapeutic levels of, 6–7
    transport of, while traveling, 23
    unintended effects of, 8, 9
antibodies, 72
anticonvulsants, 258–261, 263–264, 268–272
antidepressants, 265–266
antidiarrheals, 122–123
antiemetics, 119
antifungals, 204–206, 253
antigens, 72
antihistamines, 150–152
    accidental ingestion of, 148
    for allergic rhinitis, 143
    for behavioral control, 264–265
    for bronchitis, 145
    for colds, 147
    for eczema, 192
    for menstrual discomfort, 235–236
antiinflammatories, 206–207
antiparasitics, 203–204
antipyretics, 229, 230
antiseptics, 200–202
antitoxins, 72–73

Anti-Tuss, 155
antitussives
  for bronchitis, 145
  for colds, 147
appendicitis, laxatives and, 125
appetite suppressants, 215–216
Aqua-Mephyton, 105
Aquasol A, 97
Aquasol E, 105
Aqu-Ban, 233
Aristotle, 178
arms, swelling of, 97
arthritis
  aspirin for, 7
  vitamins and, 103
Arthropan, 88
artificial sweeteners, 10, 217–218
A.S.A., 90, 230
Ascriptin, 88, 90, 230
aspartame, 218
Aspergum, 88, 90, 230
aspirin (acetylsalicylic acid), 83, 88, 90–92
  for arthritis, 7
  fetus affected by, 10, 11
  for fever, 87, 90
  for inflammation, 89, 90
  for menstrual discomfort, 230–232
  for pain, 88–89, 90
  in pregnancy, 11, 90, 91, 230
  therapeutic levels of, 7
  vitamin C and, 103
Aspirin Free Anacin, 89, 229
asthma, 143–144
  albuterol for, 273
  bronchodilators for, 144
  cromolyn for, 275
  metaproterenol for, 279
  terbutaline for, 282–283
  theophylline for, 283–284
Atarax, 264
athlete's foot, 196, 204–206
attention deficit disorder. *See* ADD
A-200, 203
Augmentin, 240
Ayds AM/PM, 215

Bab-Eze, 209
Baciguent, 199
bacitracin, 199
Bactrim, 245
Balmex, 209
Barbital, 268
Baximim, 199
Bayer Children's Cold Tablets, 158
Bayer Decongestant, 158
Bayfrin, 156
Baytussin, 155
Baytussin AC, 152

B-Balm, 209
bed-wetting, 265–266
Beepan-VK, 254
behavioral control, medicines for, 258–272
Bell/ans, 135
Benadryl, 154, 202
Benadyne Ear Drops Improved, 185
Bendectin, 10
benzalkonium, 202, 227
benzethonium chloride, 227
benzocaine, 202, 211
benzoyl peroxide, 197
Betadine, 201
Betalin S, 98
Betapen-BK, 254
Bethaprim, 245
Bewon, 98
biliary tract, 115
bisacodyl, 126
Bisco-Lax, 126
bismuth subsalicylate, 122
Black-Draught, 134
bladder tumors, 218
bleeding
  aspirin and, 90–91
  disorders, 111, 113, 231
  vitamins and, 103, 106
blepharitis, 168, 177
Blinx, 176
Block Out, 211
boils, 246
bones
  defective growth of, 104
  deformities of, 107
  degenerative changes in, 103
  infections of, 242, 244
  vitamin A and, 97
Borax, 189
Brazelton, T. Berry, 164
breast-feeding, 11–12
  aspirin and, 91
  immunities produced by, 74
breathing difficulties, 141–159
  aspirin and, 90–91
  talcum powder and, 209
Breonesin, 155
Brethine, 282
Bricanyl, 282
Bristamycin, 249
Bromo-Seltzer, 89, 229
brompheniramine, 143, 150
bronchi, 142–143
bronchioles, 141–143
bronchiolitis, 144–145
bronchitis, 145
bronchodilators, 273, 279, 282, 283
  for asthma, 144
  nebulizers for, 60

bronchospasmolytics, 275–276
Bronkodyl, 283
Buf, 197
Bufferin, 88, 90, 230
Bu-Lax 100, 127
bulimia, 118, 215
bulk producers, 216–217

caffeine
    breast-feeding and, 11
    as diuretic, 233–234
    effects of, 216
    fetus affected by, 10
Caladryl, 202
calamine lotion, 192, 195, 202–203
Calcidrine, 152
Calciferol, 103
calcium, 106–107
calcium carbonate, 136
calcium deposits, 104
Caldecort, 206
Caldesene, 209
Camalox, 135
Ca-Plus, 106
capsules
    administration of, 33–36
    for infants, 38
    storage of, 19
    for toddlers, 40
    transport of, while traveling, 23
carbamazepine, 258
carbamide peroxide, 185
carbonic anhydrase inhibitor, 210
Cardui, 234
Casafru, 134
castor oil, 127
Ceclor, 241
cefaclor, 242–243, 247–248, 255
Cenadex, 215
Cenafed, 159
Cenagesic, 151
Cenalax, 126
Cen-E, 105
cephalexin, 243–244, 247–248, 255
cervix, 222
Cetro-Cirose, 152
Cevalin, 102
Cevita, 102
chalazions, 169
Chap Stick Sunblock 15, 211
charcoal, activated, 138–139
Charcodate, 138
Cheracol D, 153
chickenpox, 191–192
    Reye's syndrome and, 91, 231
children (two- to twelve-year-olds)
    constipation in, 124–125
    diarrhea in, 121

    skin disorders of, 191–195
    vomiting by, 117–118
Children's Aspirin, 88
Children's Tylenol, 88
Chlo-Amine, 150
chloramphenicol, 244–245
Chlor-Niramine, 150
Chloromycetin, 244
chlorothiazide, 274–275
chlorpheniramine, 143, 150–151
Chlortrimeton, 150
choking
    nosedrops and, 58
    during vomiting, 117
cholera, 79
Chooz, 136
cilia, 141
Citrate of Magnesia, 129
Citroma, 129
Citro-Nesia, 129
classification of medicines, 14
cleaning agents, 60, 200–201
Clear & Brite, 175
Clearasil, 198
Clear Eyes, 173
Clinicort, 206
clitoris, 220
clonazepam, 259–261
    medicines interacting with, 259, 260, 272
Clonopin, 259
cloxacillin, 241, 246–247, 255
Cloxapen, 246
Cluoral, 108
codeine, 152–153, 261
    for coughing, 152–153
    medicines interacting with, 124, 217, 261
    for pain, 89
Codimal DM, 153
Codylax, 126
Colace, 127
colds, 83, 87, 145–147
    vitamin C and, 103
colitis, 121, 124
Coloctyl, 127
Colrex, 153, 155
Comfolax, 127
Comfortine, 209
conjunctivitis, 167–168, 177
Consotuss, 153
constipation, 115, 124–135. *See also*
    laxatives
    in adolescents, 125
    in children, 124–125
    in infants, 124
Contac, 158
contact lenses, 169
controlled substances, 17, 258
Coppertone Shade, 211

Coricidin D, 158
Coricidin Nasal Mist, 157
corneal edema, 173
cornstarch, 207–208
Corrective Mixture, 122
Corrective Mixture w/Paregoric, 123
Correctol, 132
Cortaid, 206
corticosteroids
    for eczema, 192
    for poisonous plant irritations, 195
Cortif, 206
Coryban-D, 153, 158
Cosanyl DM Improved Formula, 153
Cotrim, 245
cotrimoxazole, 245–246
Cotussis, 152
Co-Tylenol, 89, 229
coughing
    albuterol for, 273–274
    bronchiolitis and, 145
    bronchitis and, 145
    codeine for, 152–153
    cromolyn for, 275–276
    croup and, 147
    dextromethorphan for, 153–154
    diphenhydramine for, 154–155
    guaifenesin for, 155–156
    metaproterenol for, 279–280
    terbutaline for, 282–283
    theophylline for, 283–284
Covanamine, 151
cradle cap, 190
Creamalin, 135
cromolyn, 275–276
croup, 147
Cruex, 205
Cyclopar, 256
Cylert, 267

Dalfatol, 105
D-Alpha-E, 105
Datril, 88, 89, 229
Debrox, 185
Decongestant-P, 158
decongestants, 156–159
    for allergic rhinitis, 143
    for colds, 146–147
    for otitis media, 183
Decriose, 176
Deficol, 126
Degest 2, 173
Delcid, 135
Deltalin, 103
dental caries, 108
dental fluorosis, 108
Depakene, 271
depressants, 148

DES (diethylstilbestrol), 10
Desenex, 205
Desitin, 209
Dexatrim, 215
Dexedrine, 262
dextroamphetamine, 103, 262–263
dextromethorphan, 153–154
diabetes
    insulin for, 7
    medicine ingredients and, 32
    oxymetazoline and, 157
    propranolol and, 280
    valproic acid and, 272
    weight and, 213
Diabismul, 123
Diachlor, 274
Dialume, 136
Diapa-Care Baby Powder, 207
Diaperene BP, 207
diaper rash, 189–190
    products for, 207–210
diaphragm, 143
diarrhea, 115, 119–124
    bismuth subsalicylate for, 122
    in children, 121
    chronic, 121–122
    cotrimoxazole for, 246
    gradual onset of, 120
    in infants, 119–121
    kaolin pectin for, 122–123
    laxatives and, 121
    opiates for, 123–124
    sudden onset of, 120
    treatment for, 121
Dia-Zuel, 123
Dicarbosil, 136
dicloxacillin, 241, 247–248, 255
Diet-Aid, 216
Diet-Trim, 215
Di Gel, 135
digestive system, 114–115, 116
digoxin, 276–277
    medicines interacting with, 278, 280, 282
Dilantin, 269
dimenhydrinate, 119
Dimentabs, 119
Dimetane, 150
Diosuccin, 127
Dio-Sul, 127
dioxybenzone, 210–211
Di-Phen, 269
diphenhydramine, 154–155
Di-Phenylan, 269
diphtheria, 74
    immunizations for, 72, 74, 75
Disonate, 127
Ditan, 269

diuretics, 233–235, 274, 278, 281. *See also* caffeine
  medicines interacting with, 277
Diuril, 274
DMSO (dimethyl sulfoxide), 189
Docusate Sodium, 127
Dolatoc, 127
Donnagel-PG, 123
Doxinate, 127
Dramamine, 119
Dri-Ear, 185
Drisdol, 103
Dristan Long Lasting, 156
drooling, 148
dry eye, 170
DSS (dioctyl sodium sulfosuccinate), 127–128
DTP (diphtheria, tetanus, pertussis) vaccine, 74–75
  unintended effects of, 75
Duadacin, 151
Dulcolax, 126
Dumebro, 185
Duosol, 127
Duramist Plus, 156
Duration, 156
Duration Mild, 157
Dycill, 247
Dynapen, 247
dysmenorrhea, 226

ears, 178–186
  administering medicines to, 55–57
  aluminum acetate for, 185–186
  anatomy of, 178–180
  carbamide peroxide for, 185
  external, 178–179
  foreign objects in, 181
  infections of, 78, 87, 182–184
  inner, 180
  insects in, 182
  middle, 179–180
  ringing in, 91
Eclipse, 211
Ecotrin, 90, 230
eczema, 60, 143, 192–193
  shampoos for, 61
E.E.S., 249
E-Ferol, 105
Eldodram, 119
Elecal, 106
electrolytes
  medicines and, 127, 129, 132, 133
  vomiting and, 117, 118
Elixicon, 283
elixirs, 31, 37–38
Elixophyllin, 283
emetics, 140
Empirin, 90, 230

Emulsoil, 127
E Mycin, 249
Encaprin, 90, 230
encephalitis, 76
endometrium, 222, 224
enemas, 43
enuresis, 265–266
enzyme deficiencies, 214
Epi-Clear, 197, 198
epidemic keratoconjunctivitis, 167–168
epiglottis, 148
epiglottitis, 148
  amoxicillin for, 240–241
  chloramphenicol for, 244–245
epilepsy, 6–7
Eprolin, 105
Epsilan-M, 105
Equal, 218
Equilet, 136
Ery-Ped, 249
Ery-Tab, 249
Erythrocin, 249
erythromycin, 249
  medicines interacting with, 284
esophagus, 114, 142
Estomul, 135
Estomul-M, 135
estrogen, 223
ethosuximide, 263–264
Eugel, 135
Evac-U-Lax, 132
Excedrin, 89, 229
excretion of medicines, 7–8
Ex-Lax, 132
expectorants, 155–156
expiration dates, 15, 238
Exzit, 198
Eye Cool, 174
eyes, 160–177
  administering medicines to, 48–55
  anatomy of, 160–162
  chemical injuries to, 166–167
  development of, 163–164
  dryness of, 97, 170
  foreign bodies in, 165–166
  infections of, 167–168, 177
  inflammations of, 145, 173
  injuries to, 165–166
  irrigants for, 176–177
  irritation of, 173
  medicines for, 171–176
  sun injuries to, 167
  vitamin A and, 97
Eye-Stream, 176

face
  bluish-gray, 147
  sores on, 99
fallopian tubes, 222

Federal Controlled Substances Act, 258
Feen-a-Mint, 132
Feen-a-Mint Gum, 132
feet
  cold, 147
  numbness of, 101, 102
  swelling of, 98, 105
feminine hygiene sprays, 227–228
Feosol, 108
Fergon, 110
Fer-In-Sol, 110
Ferrous Fumarate, 110
Ferrous Gluconate, 110
Ferrous Sulfate, 110
Fiberall, 216
Flacid, 135
Flagyl, 251
Flavorcee, 102
Fleet Babylax, 128
Fleet Bisacodyl, 126
Florical, 106
Flowaway Water 100's, 233
flu, 146
fluoride, 108–110
Fluorigard, 108
Fluorinse, 108
Flura, 108
Flura-Drops, 108
Flura-Loz, 108
Fluritab, 108
folic acid, 102, 270
follicles, 224
Food and Drug Administration, U.S., 96,
  155, 218, 237
food poisoning, 117–118, 121
forehead, bulging of, 97
Formula 44-D, 153
Fostex Cake, 197
FSH (follicle stimulation hormone), 224
Fulvicin P/G, 250
Fulvicin U/F, 250
fungal infections, 204–206
Furacin, 199
Furadantin, 252
Furalan, 252
Furan, 252
Furante, 252
Furatoin, 252
furosemide, 210, 278–279

gall bladder disorders, 118
Gantrisin, 256
gastroenteritis, 121
Gaviscon, 135
Gaviscon-2, 135
Gee-Gee, 154
Gelusil, 135
generic medicines
  absorption of, 5

aspirin as, 91
  requesting of, 18
generic names
  definition of, 14
  on labels, 14, 16–17
GG-Cen, 155
GG-Tussin, 155
Ginsopan, 151
glaucoma, 174–176
Glycate, 106
glycerin
  for constipation, 128–129
  for ear wax removal, 185
Glycotuss, 155
Glydeine, 152
Glytuss, 155
gonadotropin, 223
gramicidin, 199
Grifulvin V, 250
griseofulvin, 250
G-200, 155
guaifenesin, 155–156
Guiamid A.C., 152
gums, swelling of, 103

Haemophilus influenzae type B, 78
  immunizations for, 74, 78
hair, applying medicines to, 60–65
hallucinations, vitamins and, 100, 102
Halotussin w/Codeine, 152
hands
  cold, 147
  numbness of, 101, 102
  swelling of, 98, 105
hay fever, 150
heartburn, 136
heart disease
  chlorothiazide for, 274–275
  digoxin for, 276–277
  furosemide for, 278–279
  propranolol for, 280–281
  spironolactone for, 281–282
heart rhythm regulators, 280–281
heart stimulants, 276–277
Henotal, 268
hepatitis, 118
Hexa-Betalin, 101
hexachlorophene, 189, 227
histamines, 144
Hodgkin's disease, 78
Hold, 153
hookworm, 251
hordeolums, 169, 177
Hycort, 206
Hydrocil, 134
hydrocortisone, 195, 206–207
hydroxyethylcellulose, 171
hydroxypropyl methylcellulose, 171
hydroxyzine, 264–265

hyperactivity
  dextroamphetamine for, 262
  methylphenidate for, 266–267
  pemoline for, 267–268
hypercalcemia, 104, 107
hyperphosphatemia, 104
hypervitaminosis A, 97–98
hypothalamus, 223–224
Hytuss, 155
Hytuss-2X, 155

ibuprofen, 92–93
  for inflammation, 89
  for menstrual discomfort, 232–233
illicit drugs
  adolescents and, 42
  medicines interacting with, 30, 42
Ilosone, 249
Ilotycin, 249
Imavate, 265
imipramine, 124, 265–266
  drugs interacting with, 103, 265
  vitamins and, 103, 265
immune deficiency, 78
immune serum globulins, 72–73
immunizations, 71–79
  mechanism of, 72–74
  precautions taken with, 71, 75, 79
  records of, 20–21, 72, 73
  schedules for, 74
  types of, 72–73
  unintended effects of, 71
immunosuppressants, 71
impetigo, 194, 246
Inderal, 280
indigestion, 115
Infantol Pink, 123
infants (newborns to two-year-olds)
  administering medicines to, 27, 37–40
  capsules for, 38, 40
  constipation in, 124
  diarrhea in, 119–121
  eardrops for, 56
  eye medicines for, 52–53
  intravenous infusions for, 4
  kidney function in, 7–8
  liquid medicines for, 37–39
  medicine absorption in, 4–5
  medicine excretion in, 7–8
  nosedrops for, 58, 59
  rashes in, 5
  skin disorders of, 5, 188–191, 193
  skin medicines for, 63, 64
  suppositories for, 45–47
  tablets for, 40
  urination of, 8
  vitamins and, 94, 101, 102, 105, 106
  vomiting by, 115–117

inflammation, 89
  acetaminophen for, 89–90
  aspirin for, 90–91
  hydrocortisone for, 206–207
  ibuprofen for, 92–93
inflammatory bowel disease, 121, 124
influenza
  colds confused with, 146
  immunizations for, 79
  Reye's syndrome and, 91
insect bites, 202, 206
insomnia, 100
insulin, 7
Intal, 275
intestinal obstructions, 134, 217
intestinal wall
  castor oil and, 127
  mineral oil and, 131
  opiates and, 123
  phenolphthalein and, 132
iodophors, 201
ipecac, syrup of, 138–140
irritable bowel syndrome, 134
Isodine, 201
Isopto Alkaline, 171
Isopto-Frin, 174
Isopto Plain, 171
Ivarest, 202

Janimine, 265
jock itch, 204–206
Johnson & Johnson Cornstarch Baby
    Powder, 207
Johnson & Johnson Medicated Powder, 208,
    209
Johnson Baby Powder, 208
joint pain, 97

Kaodene #1, 123
Kaodene #2, 123
Kaodonna PG, 123
kaolin pectin, 122–123
Kaolin w/Pectin, 122
Kaomead, 122
Kaomead PG, 123
Kaopectate, 122
Kapectolin PG, 123
Kappadione, 105
Kaybovite, 101
Keflex, 243
Kellogg's Castor Oil, 127
keratolytic drugs, 197–199
Kobac, 123
Kodet SE, 159
Kolantyl, 135
Kondremul Plain, 131
K-P, 122
Kudrox, 135

labels, 13–17
   on nonprescription medicines, 13–15
   on prescription medicines, 15–17
labia, 220
Lacril, 171
L. A. Formula, 134
Lanoxicaps, 276
Lanoxin, 276
large intestine, 114
Larotid, 240
Lasix, 278
Lauro, 176
Lavoptik Eye Wash, 176
Laxadan Supules, 123
laxatives, 43, 125–135
learning disabilities, 96, 110
Ledercillin VK, 254
legs, swelling of, 97
LH (luteinizing hormone), 224
lice
   head, 60, 61, 193–194
   pyrethins with piperonyl butoxide for,
      203–204
lips
   bluish-gray, 147
   sores on, 99
liquid medicines
   administration of, 31–33, 37–38
   for ears, 55
   for eyes, 48–52
   for infants, 37–38
   measuring of, 32–33
   for toddlers, 40
   transportation of, 23
Liquifilm Forte, 172
Liquifilm Tears, 172
Liquiprin, 88, 89, 229
Liquitussin, 155
Liquitussin A.C., 152
Listerex, 197
liver, 115
lockjaw. *See* tetanus
lot numbers, 15
Luminal, 268
lung disease, 269
lungs, 141–142
Lyteers, 171

Maalox #1, 135
Maalox #2, 135
Maalox Plus, 135
Macrodantin, 252
Magnagel, 135
Magnatril, 135
magnesium citrate, 129–130
magnesium hydroxide, 130–131, 136
Mallamint, 136
Malotuss, 155

Marmine, 119
massage, for fever, 87
measles, 76
   colds confused with, 146
   immunizations for, 72, 74, 77, 191
mebendazole, 251
Melozets, 216
menarche, 219–224
meningitis, 78
   chloramphenicol for, 244–245
   rifampin for, 255
menstruation, 219–236
   cramps from, 83, 118
mental illness, 96
meperidine, 124, 153, 261
Mephyton, 105
merbromin, 201–202
Mercurochrome, 201
Metamucil, 134, 216
Metaprel, 279
metaproterenol, 279–280
Methopto-Forte ½%, 171
Methopto-Forte 1%, 171
Methopto ¼%, 171
methylcellulose, 171, 217
methylphenidate, 266
metronidazole, 42, 251–252
Metryl, 251
Mexsana Medicated Powder, 207
Micatin, 204
miconazole, 204–205
Midol, 233
milia, 191
Milk of Magnesia, 130, 136
Milroy Artificial Tears, 171
mineral oil, 131–132
   vitamins and, 104, 106
Mint-o-mag, 136
MMR (measles, mumps, rubella) vaccines,
   76–78
Modane Bulk, 134
Modane Soft, 127
Mongolian spots, 191
mononucleosis, 242
morphine, 124, 153, 261
Motion-Aid, 119
mouth
   dryness of, 107, 119
   soreness of, 102
   sores in, 101
M/Rinse, 176
Mucilose, 134
mumps, 76
   immunizations for, 72, 74, 77
Murine Ear Drops, 185
Murine Eye Drops, 171
Murine Plus Eye Drops, 175
Murocel Ophthalmic Solution, 171

Muro Tears, 171
muscles
    coordination of, 102
    pain in, 83, 97
    spasms of, 107
    weakness of, 98
Mychel, 244
Myciguent, 199
Mycitracin, 199
Mycostatin, 253
Mylanta, 135
Mylanta II, 135
Mylicon, 137
myringotomy tubes, 55, 182, 184–186
Mysoline, 271

naphazoline hydrochloride, 173–175
Naphcon, 173
narcotics, 261
nasal cavities, 141
Nasalcrom, 275
National Academy of Sciences, Food and
    Nutrition Board of, 94
National Research Council, 94
National Society for the Prevention of
    Blindness, 164
nebulizers, 60
Neo-Calglucon, 106
Neo-Cultol, 131
Neo-Fed, 159
Neoloid, 127
neomycin, 71, 199
Neo-Polycin, 199
Neosporin, 199
Neo-Synephrine, 157
Neosynephrine 12 Hour, 156
Neo-Synephrinol Day, 159
Nervine, 150
Neutracomp, 135
Neutralox, 135
newborns
    eye development in, 163–164
    eye problems in, 164–165
    hearing in, 178
nicotinamide, 100
Nicotinex, 100
Nicotinic Acid (Niacin), 100
Nilstat, 253
nitrofurantoin, 252–253
nonprescription medicines
    labels of, 13–15
    packaging of, 14, 18
    strengths of, 17
    understanding actions of, 17, 18
Noralac, 135
Nortussin, 155
Nortussin w/Codeine, 152

nose
    administering medicines by, 57–60
    foreign objects in, 148–149
    function of, 141–142
nosedrops
    for colds, 146
    overuse of, 146
Nostril, 157
Nostrilla, 156
Novafed, 159
Novahistine, 158
Novahistine DMX, 153
Noxzema 12-Hour Acne Medicine, 198
NP-27, 205
Nujol, 131
Nuprin, 92, 232
Nutrasweet, 218
Nuvac, 123
Nyquil, 153
nystatin, 32, 253–254
Nytol, 150

Odrinex, 215
Odrinil, 233
Omnipen, 241
opiates, 123–124, 217, 261
Optigene II Eye Drops, 174
Optigene III, 175
oral suspensions, 31–32
Orazinc, 112
Ornex, 158
Oscal 500, 106
otitis externa, 182–183
otitis media, 78, 183–184
    amoxicillin for, 240–241
    cephalexin for, 243–244
    chloramphenicol for, 244–245
    colds confused with, 146
    sulfisoxazole for, 256
ovaries, 222, 224
overweight, 213–214. *See also* weight control
oxybenzone, 211–212
Oxy 5, 197
oxymetazoline, 156

PABA (p-aminobenzoic acid), 210–211
Pabagel, 210
Pabanol, 210
Pabizol with Paregoric, 123
pamabrom, 234–235
Pamprin, 234, 235
Panadol, 88, 89, 229
Pan-B-1, 98
Pan-B-6, 101
pancreas, 115
Panmycin, 256

parasitic infections, 251
  pyrethins with piperonyl butoxide for, 203–204
Parelixir, 123
Pargel, 122
Parsadox, 197
passive immunity, 73
Pathocil, 247
Pediaflor, 108
Pediamycin, 249
pediculosis, 193–194
pemoline, 267–268
Penapar VK, 254
penicillin, 254–255
  allergies to, 9, 241, 243, 249, 250
Pentids, 254
Pen-Vee K, 254
Pepto-Bismol, 122
periorbital cellulitis, 245
Pernox, 197
Pertussin 8-Hour, 153
pertussis, 75
  colds confused with, 146
  immunizations for, 72, 74, 75
Petrogalar Plain, 131
petrolatum, 208
P.E. (polyethylene myringotomy) tubes, 55, 182, 184–186
Pfizer E, 249
Pfizerpen-A, 241
Pfizerpen VK, 254
pharnyx, 141–142
Phenaphen, 88, 89, 229
phenobarbital, 6–7
  medicines interacting with, 259, 269, 270, 272, 284
  for seizure control, 6–7, 268–269
  vitamin D and, 104
Phenolax, 132
phenolphthalein, 132–133
phenylephrine, 157–158
phenylpropanolamine, 158–159
  in "speed," 42, 159, 216
  for weight control, 215–216
Phenylzin, 174
phenytoin
  medicines interacting with, 270, 272
  for seizure control, 269–271
  vitamin D and, 104
Phenytoin Sodium, 269
pHiso Ac, 198
phosphosoda, 133–134
P.H. Tabs, 136
pinworm, 251
piperonyl butoxide, 203–204
pituitary gland, 223–224
PKU (phenylketonuria), 218

pleura, 143
PMS (premenstrual syndrome), 226–227, 233, 236
pneumonia, 78
  amoxicillin for, 240–241
  cephalexin for, 243–244
pneumonitis, 131
poisoning
  activated charcoal for, 138–139
  syrup of ipecac for, 139–140
poisonous plants, 194–195
  calamine for, 202–203
polio, 76
  oral vaccine for, 72, 74, 76
Polycillin, 241
Polycin, 199
polymixin, 199
Polymox, 240
Polysporin, 199
polyvinyl alcohol, 172–173
Poviderm, 201
Prefrin Liquifilm, 174
pregnancy, 10–11
  aspirin during, 11, 90, 91, 230
  ibuprofen during, 92
  immunizations during, 71, 79
  iron during, 111
  MMR vaccine during, 77
  rubella during, 76
Presamine, 265
preschoolers (three- to six-year-olds)
  administering medicines to, 28–29, 40
  eardrops for, 57
  eye medicines for, 54
  nosedrops for, 59
  skin medicines for, 63–64
  skin of, 5
  suppositories for, 47–48
  urination of, 8
  wound treatments for, 63–64
prescription number, 16
PreSun, 210
prickly heat, 191
primidone, 271
Principen, 241
progesterone, 224
Propadrine, 158, 215
Propagest, 158
propranolol, 280–281
Protostat, 251
Proventil, 273
Prulet, 132
pseudoephedrine, 159
psyllium seed, 134, 217
puberty, 29–30, 219–220
Purge, 127
pyloric stenosis, 10

pylorus, 114
pyrethins with piperonyl butoxide, 203–204
Pyridoxine, 101
pyrilamine, 151–152
pyrilamine maleate, 235–236

Quinsana Plus, 205

rabies, vaccine for, 79
R&C, 203
Recommended Daily Allowances (RDAs),
    94–96, 97
records, 20–22
rectal sphincter, 221
rectum, 44
Redisol, 101
Regacilium, 134
Reguloid, 134
Regutol, 127
Relax-U, 151
respiration, depressed, 110
Res-Q, 138
retinoic acid
    for acne, 98
    oral vitamin A vs., 98
Reye's syndrome, 91, 231
Rhindecon, 158, 215
rhinitis, allergic, 143
rickets, 104
Rid, 203
Rifadin, 255
rifampin, 255–256
Rimactane, 255
ringworm, 195, 204–206
Riopan Plus, 135
Ritalin, 266
Robicillin VK, 254
Robinmycin, 249
Robitet, 256
Robitussin, 155
Robitussin A-C, 152
Robitussin DM, 153
Rocky Mountain spotted fever, 195
Rolaids, 135
Romilar Children's, 153
rubella, 76
    blood test for, 77–78
    immunizations for, 72, 74, 77, 191
RV Paba Stick, 210

saccharin, 217–218
St. Joseph's Cold Tablets for Children, 158
St. Joseph's Cough Syrup for Children, 153
salicylic acid, 197–198
Saligel Acne Gel, 197
saliva, excessive, 100
sanitary napkins, 228

Satric, 251
school-agers (six- to twelve-year-olds)
    administering medicines to, 29, 41–42
    eardrops for, 57
    eye medicines for, 55
    nosedrops for, 59
    skin medicines for, 64–65
    skin of, 5
    suppositories for, 48
    wound treatment for, 64–65
scurvy, 103
seborrhea, 190
sedatives, 268–269
    accidental ingestion of, 148
seizures
    calcium and, 107
    carbamazepine for, 258–259
    clonazepam for, 259–261
    in epileptics, 6
    ethosuximide for, 263–264
    fluoride and, 108
    increasing frequency of, 260, 263
    phenobarbital for, 6–7, 268–269
    phenytoin for, 269–270
    primidone for, 271
    valproic acid, 271–272
senna extract, 134–135
Senokot, 134
Septra, 245
Serutan, 216
shampoos, 61–62
Siblin, 134
sickle cell disease, 78
Silain-Gel, 135
Simaal Gel, 135
Simeco, 135
simethicone, 137
Sinarest Nasal, 157
Sine-Off, 158
Sinex, 157
Sinex Long-Lasting, 156
Sinurex, 158
sinusitis, 149
    amoxicillin for, 240–241
    cotrimoxazole for, 245–246
Sinustate, 158
Sinutab, 158
SK-Ampicillin, 241
SK-Bisacodyl, 126
SK-Chlorothiazide, 274
SK-Erythromycin, 249
SK-Furosemide, 278
skin, 5, 187–212
    adolescent disorders of, 195–196
    anatomy of, 187–188
    applying medicines to, 60–65
    childhood disorders of, 191–195

skin *(cont.)*
  dry, 190
  functions of, 187
  infant disorders of, 188–191, 193
  infections of, 242, 244, 250
  medicines for, 5, 197–212
SK-Niacin, 100
SK-Penicillin VK, 254
SK-Phenobarbital, 268
SK-Pramine, 265
SK-Soxazole, 256
SK-Terpin Hydrate and Codeine, 152
SK-Tetracycline, 256
Slo-bid, 283
Slo-Phyllin, 283
small intestine, 114
smallpox, 71, 79
smell, impaired, 112
SMZ-TMP, 245
Soda-Mint, 136
sodium bicarbonate, 136–137
Solar Cream, 210
Solucap E, 105
Sominex, 151
Somophyllin-T, 283
Soothe Eye Drops, 174, 175
sore throats, antihistamines and, 147
Span-Niacin-150, 100
Spantrol, 215
Spectrocin, 199
Spec-T Sore Throat/Cough Suppressant, 153
"speed," 42, 159, 216
spironolactone, 281–282
spitting up, 115–117
staphylococcus aureus, 227
S-T Expectorant, 155
stimulants, 262–263, 266
stomach, 114
stools
  black, 110
  blood in, 120, 124
  hard, 9
storage of medicines, 18–20
Stulex, 127
styes, 169, 177
Sucaryl, 217
Sudafed, 159
Sudrin, 159
sulfa-containing medicines, 9
Sulfatrim, 245
sulfisoxazole, 256
sulfonamides, 210–211
sulfonylurea, 210
Sulforcin, 198
sulfur, 198–199
Sumox, 240
Sumycin, 256

sunburn, 202
Sundown, 211
Sunril, 234, 235
sunscreens, 210–212
Super Anahist, 158
superinfections, 239
suppositories, 43–48
  for adolescents, 48
  for infants, 45–47
  for preschoolers, 47–48
  for school-agers, 48
  for toddlers, 47
Sust-A, 97
swallowing, painful, 148
Sweeta, 217
swimmer's ear, 182–183
Syllact, 134
Synkavite, 105

tablets
  administration of, 33–36
  for infants, 40
  for toddlers, 40
talcum powder, 208–209
tampons, 67, 227, 229
taste, impaired, 112
Tear-efrin Eye Drops, 174
Tearisol, 171
Tears Plus, 172
Tegopen, 246
Tegretol, 258
Teldrin, 150
Tempra, 88, 89, 229
terbutaline, 282–283
Terpin Hydrate w/Codeine, 152
tetanus, 74–75
  immunizations for, 72, 74, 75
Tetrachel, 256
tetracycline, 256–257
  for acne, 196, 199
  fetus affected by, 10
  minerals interacting with, 107, 111, 112
Tetracyn, 256
tetrahydrozoline hydrochloride, 175–176
Tetrasine, 175
TexSix T.R., 101
thalidomide, 10
Theobid, 283
Theo-Dur, 283
Theolair, 283
Theophyl, 283
theophylline, 283–284
Thera-Flur, 108
Theralax, 126
therapeutic levels, 5–7
  administration schedules and, 6–7
  body fat and, 6

therapeutic levels *(cont.)*
  body surface area and, 5–6
  definition of, 5, 8
thermometers, 84–87
  electronic, 84
  oral vs. rectal, 84
thiazide diuretic, 210
thrush, 32, 253
thyroid excess, 214
ticks, 195
Tinactin, 205
Tinea capitis, 195
Tinea corpus, 195
tobacco smoke, fetus affected by, 10
Tocopher-M, 105
toddlers (one- to three-year-olds)
  administering medicines to, 27–28, 40
  capsules for, 40
  eardrops for, 56
  eye medicines for, 53–54
  liquid medicines for, 40
  nosedrops for, 58
  skin medicines for, 63
  suppositories for, 47
  urination of, 8
  wound treatment for, 63
Tofranil, 265
tolnaftate, 205
Tolu-Sed, 152
tongue
  sores on, 99, 101
  swollen, 100
tonsillectomies, 91
TOPV (trivalent oral polio vaccine), 74, 76
Totacillin, 241
toxoids, 72. *See also* immunizations
trachea, 141–143
  foreign bodies in, 149
trade names
  definition of, 14
  on labels, 14, 16–17
  misleading nature of, 17
Transact, 198
transportation of medicines, 23–24
Trav-Arex, 119
Trendar, 234, 235
Trialka, 135
Triaminic, 158
Triaminicin, 158
Triaminicol, 153
Tri-Aqua, 233
trichomoniasis, 251
trimethoprim-sulfa, 245–246
Trimox, 240
Triple Antibiotic Ointment, 199
Triplex, 203
Trisogel, 135
Trisol Eye Wash, 176

Tritralac, 135
TSS (toxic shock syndrome), 227, 229
tuberculosis
  rifampin for, 255
  testing for, 79
Tums, 136
2/G, 155
2/G-DM, 153
Tylenol, 89, 229
typhoid, immunizations for, 79

ulcers
  aspirin and, 90, 230
  bleeding, 126
Ultra Tears, 171
undeclyenic acid, 205–206
underweight, 214–215
urethral opening, 220–221
urinary tract infections
  amoxicillin for, 240–241
  cefaclor for, 242–243
  cephalexin for, 243–244
  cotrimoxazole for, 245–246
  nitrofurantoin for, 252–253
  sulfisoxazole for, 256
urination, 8
  phenolphthalein and, 133
U.S. Food and Drug Administration, 96,
    155, 218, 237
uterus, 222, 224
Utimox, 240

vaccines, 72. *See also* immunizations
Vacon, 157
vagina, 221–222
  applying medicines to, 65–67
  douches for, 228
  infections of, 42
vaginal adenocarcinoma, 10
Valihist, 151
valproic acid, 271–272
  medicines interacting with, 259, 260
Vanoxide, 197
Vaseline Pure Petroleum Jelly, 208
Vaso-Clear, 173
Ventilade, 151
Ventolin, 273
Veracillin, 247
Vermox, 251
Vertiban, 119
Vicks, 153
Vicks Formula-44 Cough Discs, 153
Visculose-1%, 171
Visine, 175
Visine A.C., 175
vision, vitamins and, 99, 102
Vistaril, 264
Vitacee, 102

vitamin A, 97–98
  for acne, 98, 196
vitamin B₁ (thiamine), 98–99
vitamin B₂ (riboflavin), 99
vitamin B₃ (nicotinic acid or niacin), 100
vitamin B₆ (pyridoxine), 101
  premenstrual syndrome and, 236
vitamin B₁₂ (cyanocobalamine), 101–102
vitamin C (ascorbic acid), 102–103
vitamin D (ergocalciferol), 103–104
vitamin E, 105
vitamin K, 105–106
vitamins, 94–106
  definition of, 94
  excessive intake of, 96–97
  mineral oil and, 131
  recommended intake of, 95
  therapeutic levels of, 6
Vita-Plus E, 105
Vita-Slim, 215
Viterra C, 102
V-Lax, 134
vomiting
  by adolescents, 118
  chemical ingestion and, 118
  by children, 118
  dimenhydrinate for, 119
  by infants, 115–117
  spitting up vs., 115–117

warnings, on labels, 15, 17
weight control, 213–218
  aspartame for, 218
  bulk producers for, 216–217
  phenylpropanolamine for, 216–217
  saccharin for, 217–218
welts, 120
whipworm, 251
whooping cough. *See* pertussis
Win-Gel, 135
wounds, 61–64, 103, 113
Wyamycin E, 249
Wymox, 240

X-Prep, 127

yeast infections, 242–244, 253
yellow fever, immunizations for, 79

Zarontin, 263
zinc, 112–113
Zincate, 112
Zincfrin, 174
Zinc Gluconate, 112
zinc oxide, 209–210
Zinc Sulfate, 112
Zinkaps-110, 112
ZNG, 112
Zn-Plus, 112
Zymenol, 131

About the Authors

Ruth McGillis Bindler is an Associate Professor of Nursing at the Intercollegiate Center for Nursing Education in Spokane, Washington. She earned a Bachelor of Science in Nursing from Cornell University and a Master of Science in Child Development from the University of Wisconsin. She currently resides in Washington.

Yvonne Tso practiced as a clinical pharmacist at Children's Orthopedic Hospital and Medical Center after graduating from the University of Washington. She has also worked as a consultant in the Seattle Regional Poison Control Center. She now lives and works in California.

Linda Berner Howry earned a Bachelor of Science in Nursing from Northern Illinois University and a Master of Science from the University of Colorado. Formerly an assistant professor at the Intercollegiate Center for Nursing Education in Spokane, Washington, she now resides in California.